PSYCHOSOCIAL NURSING CONCEPTS

An Activity Book

THIRD EDITION

PSYCHOSOCIAL NURSING CONCEPTS

An Activity Book

THIRD EDITION

HOLLY SKODOL WILSON
RN, PhD, FAAN

CAROL REN KNEISL
RN, MS

ADDISON-WESLEY PUBLISHING COMPANY
Health Sciences Division, Menlo Park, California
Reading, Massachusetts • Menlo Park, California • New York
Don Mills, Ontario • Wokingham, England • Amsterdam • Bonn
Sydney • Singapore • Tokyo • Madrid • Bogota • Santiago • San Juan

Sponsoring Editor: Tracy L. Corral
Production Management: Michael Bass & Associates

ISBN 0-201-11895-5
ABCDEFGHIJ-BA-891098

Addison-Wesley Publishing Company
Health Sciences Division
2725 Sand Hill Road
Menlo Park, California 94025

PREFACE

Since the publication of the first edition of this book, nursing instructors and their students have enthusiastically welcomed it as a learning resource. Originally designed to combine the varied and many guides to teaching psychiatric nursing, the third edition also continues this tradition. Our goal for the workbook was to fill a need and enliven important concepts, theories, and skills for students and faculty alike. Educators have used *Psychosocial Nursing Concepts: An Activity Book* to supplement instruction in specific courses such as nursing fundamentals, community health, and leadership, as well as in integrated programs where it is used throughout the nursing curriculum.

This workbook is one element of a three-part set. The three components—workbook, testbank, and text—form a complete package for teaching theoretical and clinical psychiatric nursing, either as a separate course or as an integrated part of a nursing curriculum. It can also be used as a stand-alone book in conjunction with *any* psychiatric nursing text.

FEATURES

This workbook contains the following to help the student make the connection between theory and practice:

Individual and small group exercises

Inventories and questionnaires

Assessment tools

Simulations

By using this workbook, students live through and experience the interpersonal relationships they have read about. Additionally, they learn about values and how their values influence nursing care, and how personal attributes influence the role of each nurse.

ORGANIZATION

Students and faculty alike will find a wide array of classroom and clinical tools within *Psychosocial Nursing Concepts: An Activity Book*. Part One focuses attention on the psychosocial nurse as a person. The learning activities in this part concern the person-as-nurse relationships and experiences in nursing practice. Part Two presents assessment exercises in addition to learning activities that deal with psychosocial nursing interventions. These assessment exercises encourage the nurse to solve problems and make decisions based on systematically collecting data, rather than using preconceived interpretations or the experiences of others. The interventions activities provide simulated situations, directions, and a structured format for feedback and interaction with peers and faculty.

ACKNOWLEDGEMENTS

This third edition reflects the help we have received from nursing faculty and nursing students in the United States and Canada, who took time from their busy lives to make suggestions and to request additions. We have carefully reviewed each and every comment. To encourage even more readers to share their experiences of this text, we have included a self-addressed, stamped comment card on the last page of the book. We look forward to receiving your invaluable feedback.

H.S.W.
C.R.K.

CONTENTS

Part Two   PSYCHOSOCIAL NURSING ASSESSMENTS, STRATEGIES, AND SKILLS

Part One

THE PERSON AS
PSYCHOSOCIAL NURSE

Beliefs about "Mental Illness"

DIRECTIONS

The following statements reflect ideas and beliefs about conditions that are labeled "mental illness" and about people who become "mental patients." Rate each with a score ranging from 5 to 0, based on the following scale:

5 Strongly agree   2 Not sure but probably disagree

4 Agree   1 Disagree

3 Not sure but probably agree   0 Strongly disagree

There are no right or wrong answers, so be as honest as you can.

_____ 1. When you have a problem or worry, it is better not to think about it but rather keep busy with more pleasant things.

_____ 2. All clients in mental hospitals should be prevented by a painless operation from having children.

_____ 3. One of the main causes of mental illness is a lack of moral strength or will power.

_____ 4. Every person should have complete faith in some supernatural power whose decisions he or she obeys without question.

_____ 5. Although some mental clients seem all right, it is dangerous to forget for a moment that they are mentally ill.

_____ 6. Even though clients in mental hospitals behave in funny ways, it is wrong to laugh about them.

_____ 7. Clients in mental hospitals are in many ways like children.

Source: Copyright 1962 by the American Psychological Association. Adapted by permission of the publisher and authors. "Opinions about Mental Illness Scale," by Jacob Cohen and E. L. Struening, *Journal of Abnormal and Social Psychology* Vol. 64, No. 5, 1962, pp. 349-360.

_____ 8. Our mental hospitals seem more like prisons than like places where mentally ill people can be cared for.

_____ 9. Although they usually aren't aware of it, many people become mentally ill to avoid the difficult problems of everyday life.

_____ 10. More tax money should be spent in the care and treatment of people with severe mental illness.

_____ 11. Many mental clients are capable of skilled labor, even though in some ways they are very disturbed mentally.

_____ 12. Many people who have never been clients in a mental hospital are more mentally ill than many hospitalized mental clients.

_____ 13. Many mental clients would remain in the hospital until they were well even if the doors were unlocked.

_____ 14. The clients of a mental hospital should have something to say about the way the hospital is run.

_____ 15. More tax money should be spent in the care and treatment of people with severe mental illness.

_____ 16. A woman would be foolish to marry a man who has had a severe mental illness, even though he seems fully recovered.

_____ 17. People who have been clients in a mental hospital will never be their old selves again.

_____ 18. Small children should not be allowed to visit their parents who are clients in mental hospitals.

_____ 19. Most clients in mental hospitals don't care how they look.

_____ 20. Anyone who is in a hospital for a mental illness should not be allowed to vote.

_____ 21. Mental clients come from homes where the parents took little interest in their children.

_____ 22. The mental illness of many people is caused by the separation or divorce of their parents during childhood.

_____ 23. If parents loved their children more, there would be less mental illness.

_____ 24. If the children of normal parents were raised by mentally ill parents, they would probably become mentally ill.

_____ 25. People who are successful in their work seldom become mentally ill.

EXPLANATION OF SCORING

Five attitude orientations are represented in the above twenty-five items. Each scale is scored separately. Add your individual scores for attitude items 1-5, 6-10, 11-15, 16-20, and 21-25. Total scores for each scale can range from a high of 25 to a low of 0.

Scale A *Authoritarianism* (items 1-5). These items reflect a view of the mentally ill as an inferior class requiring coercive handling.

Scale B *Benevolence* (6-10). This scale reflects a kindly paternalistic view of patients, with emphasis on religion and humanism rather than science.

Scale C *Mental Hygiene Ideology* (11-15). This reflects an orientation that embodies the tenets of modern mental health professionals and the mental hygiene movement.

Scale D *Social Restrictiveness* (16-20). The key belief here is that mentally ill people are a threat to society, particularly the family, and therefore must be restricted in their functioning.

Scale E *Interpersonal Etiology* (21-25). This scale reflects the belief that mental illness arises from interpersonal experience, especially deprivation of parental love during childhood.

To profile your results, draw a line through each row of the chart below at the point on the row that represents your score. Shade in in the area between zero and the line you have drawn in each row.

	0	5	10	15	20	25
Scale A *Authoritarianism*						
Scale B *Benevolence*						
Scale C *Mental Hygiene Ideology*						
Scale D *Social Restrictiveness*						
Scale E *Interpersonal Etiology*						

DISCUSSION GUIDELINES

After each of you has arrived at a total score for each scale, discuss the five scales by name, considering these questions:

1. What in your own life experience might have led to the dominance of one attitude orientation or another?

2. Would you have predicted the scales on which you received high scores?

3. How might your attitudes influence your interactions and effectiveness with psychiatric clients?

4. How do terms such as *willpower, mentally ill,* etc., affect your judgment?

2

Beliefs about Psychiatric Nursing: An Ideology Scale

DIRECTIONS

The following statements reflect ideas and beliefs about psychiatric nursing and what psychiatric nurses should do in their practice. Rate each with a score ranging from 5 to 0, based on the following scale:

5 Strongly agree

4 Agree

3 Not sure but probably agree

2 Not sure but probably disagree

1 Disagree

0 Strongly disagree

_____ 1. Drugs are the most effective form of treatment for emotionally disturbed persons.

_____ 2. The psychiatric nurse should function as an agent for social change.

_____ 3. Psychiatric nurses can be more effective working indirectly with large numbers of clients than working intensively with small numbers of clients.

_____ 4. In inpatient settings, somatic forms of treatment tend to be more effective than milieu therapy or psychotherapy.

_____ 5. Working relations among members of the mental health professions would probably improve considerably if all professionals addressed each other by first name.

_____ 6. Psychotherapy reflects greater respect for the client as an individual than any other form of treatment.

_____ 7. Most hospitalized clients should be strongly encouraged to become actively involved in the treatment of other clients on their unit.

_____ 8. The psychiatric nurse is responsible for the emotionally disturbed person who does not seek the nurse out, as well as for the one who does.

_____ 9. The treatment of the mentally ill cannot be expected to improve materially until the neurological and biochemical bases for mental illness are better understood.

_____ 10. One of the main problems in mental health care is that intensive one-to-one psychotherapy is not used enough.

7

_____ 11.   Psychiatric nurses should have extensive training in the theory and findings of social psychology.

_____ 12.   Electroconvulsive therapy is the most effective treatment for severe depression.

_____ 13.   Persons in mental hospitals should be allowed to participate in deciding who among them should be discharged.

_____ 14.   Psychological factors are the most important in the etiology of mental disorder.

_____ 15.   It is unfortunate that more psychiatric nurses are not well grounded in the theories and findings of sociology and anthropology.

_____ 16.   By and large, excellence in psychiatric nursing practice requires a solid foundation in neurology.

_____ 17.   Psychiatric patients usually cannot be expected to improve their functioning significantly without slow and careful exploration of underlying psychological conflicts.

_____ 18.   The education of psychiatric nurses should emphasize understanding community mental health.

_____ 19.   Psychiatric settings should employ large numbers of nurse-psychotherapists.

_____ 20.   The inequalities that exist among mental health personnel hamper the delivery of services.

_____ 21.   Psychiatric nurses should be active in developing mental health programs for persons who are potentially vulnerable to life stresses.

_____ 22.   A serious shortcoming of milieu therapy is that it allows the client to escape establishing an intensive therapeutic relationship.

_____ 23.   A noisy and messy inpatient unit can still be a therapeutic environment.

_____ 24.   Only persons with considerable training should be allowed to form close relationships with mental clients.

_____ 25.   One of the major functions of the psychiatric nurse should be to teach clients about the medications they are receiving.

_____ 26.   Psychiatric nurses must understand their own personalities before they can be effective therapists.

_____ 27.   Treatment of hospitalized clients is most effective when the client has several close relationships with staff members rather than a single one with a therapist.

_____ 28.   An effective treatment plan for a client involves community agencies in working with the client.

_____ 29.   Team work is best accomplished when the recognized leader of the team is a psychiatrist.

_____ 30.   For the client's well-being it is important to make as accurate a diagnosis as possible.

_____ 31.   Consumers should have a strong say in the planning and operation of mental health programs.

_____ 32.   An inpatient psychiatric facility is only one part of a comprehensive mental health program for a community.

EXPLANATION OF SCORING

Four ideological orientations are represented in the above thirty-two items. Each scale is scored separately. Add your individual scores for the items listed under each scale below. Total scores for each scale can range from a high of 40 to a low of 0.

Scale A   *Medical Model Ideology* (items 1, 4, 9, 12, 16, 25, 29, 30). These items reflect a view based on an illness model that emphasizes somatic therapy.

Scale B   *Milieu Therapy Ideology* (items 5, 7, 11, 13, 15, 20, 23, 27). This scale represents the belief that the psychiatric hospital as a social system, rather than the individual, is the subject of analysis and intervention.

Scale C   *Psychotherapist/Counselor Ideology* (items 6, 10, 14, 17, 19, 22, 24, 26). This scale focuses on psychotherapy as a specific treatment for specific psychological trauma and emphasizes the individual therapist-client relationship.

Scale D   *Community Mental Health Ideology* (items 2, 3, 8, 18, 21, 28, 31, 32). These items reflect an orientation toward social action as a means of promoting mental health and the treatment of mental illness in total populations.

To profile your results, draw a line through each row of the chart below at the point on the row that represents your score. Shade in the area between zero and the line you have drawn in each row.

	0 5 10 15 20 25 30 35 40
Scale A Medical Model	
Scale B Milieu Therapy	
Scale C Psychotherapist/Counselor	
Scale D Community Mental Health	

DISCUSSION GUIDELINES

After each of you has arrived at a total score for the four ideological orientations, discuss them by name, considering such questions as:

1. What in your life and professional experience might have led to the dominance of one psychiatric nursing ideology over another?

2. Would you have predicted the scales on which you received high scores? Low scores?

3. How might your ideological orientations influence your interactions and effectiveness with psychiatric clients?

4. Which orientations do you think are humanistic in nature?

3

Are They Clients or Patients?

DIRECTIONS

In the columns below list all the words, phrases, and expressions you can think of that symbolize the words *client* and *patient*.

CLIENT	PATIENT

DISCUSSION GUIDELINES

After you have completed the two lists, compare them for similarities and differences. Then, divide into groups of five to compare your lists with those of the others in your group, considering these questions:

1. What are the major differences?
2. What are the major similarities?
3. Which words, phrases, or expressions have the most negative associations?
4. Which words, phrases, or expressions have the most positive associations?
5. How would you prefer to be treated? As a client? As a patient?
6. What nursing behaviors encourage a client role?
7. What nursing behaviors encourage a patient role?

4

Client Preference

The client is the dimension of nursing that your practice serves. The client may be an individual or a specific group. In exploring clients as individuals, identify the traits, stage, and style of persons with whom you prefer to practice. For example, in considering stage are you captured by the physical development of the young, the social complexities of the middle-aged, or the psychologic adjustments of the elderly? Does the mature person who is suddenly struck by a heart attack draw your empathy, or does the distrustful adolescent who attempts suicide evoke your healing sensitivities? Are there style dimensions that you prefer? Is it the fast-track business person or the traditional homemaker who draws your nursing interventions? Consider racial, sexual, and cultural factors, and the degree of diversity or congruence with your background and interests. Were you raised in a minority culture but now seek the challenge of dealing with diverse clients in metropolitan centers? Do you prefer to work with women as they deal with social change? Are you drawn to migrant farmers whose experiences and lifestyles are of major concern to your community?

Also think of clients in terms of groups, which are formed by family relationships, by shared health problems, or by other dimensions such as age or geography.

Complete the following statements by writing your description of client.

1. I find that I work best with clients who have the following personal traits:

   _____

   _____

2. Clients in this stage of life:

   _____

   _____

Source: Henderson FC, McGettigan BO: *Managing Your Career in Nursing* (Addison-Wesley, 1986), pp. 122–123.

3. Clients with this lifestyle:

_____

_____

4. Clients with this education or experiential background:

_____

_____

5. I work more effectively with clients in these groupings (specify individuals, small groups, organizations as a whole, or other):

_____

_____

_____

_____

6. How do preferred characteristics or groupings relate to *your* stage, style, characteristics and attributes? _____

_____

_____

_____

DISCUSSION GUIDELINES

In a group of four or five discuss your personal client preferences. Consider how your preferences might affect your psychiatric nursing practice.

5

Escape from Primavera Island: A Values Clarification Exercise

Primavera, a small island in the Pacific Ocean "ring of fire" (the circular area on the globe that contains most of the world's volcanoes and active earthquake activity), has been devastated by the unexpected eruption of an undersea volcano, which arose just off its west shore. Twelve survivors on the island have just received warning, by shortwave radio, of a *tsunami*, an oceanic tidal wave created by the unusual earthquakes and volcanic activity in this area of the Pacific. The tsunami is expected to reach Primavera in one hour. Its force and height will completely engulf and submerge the small, flat island. One helicopter has been dispatched to Primavera to rescue the survivors. Because of the distance between Primavera and other land masses, this is the only helicopter that will be able to reach it before the tsunami hits. There are no ships in the immediate area. The Sikorsky F77 helicopter can carry six passengers. Overloaded, it will probably be able to carry an absolute maximum of eight. Thus there will be room for seven passengers at the most, plus the pilot.

DIRECTIONS

Your group has only one hour to decide which seven of the twelve survivors on Primavera will escape the certain death the tsunami will bring. You must reach a decision before the tsunami reaches Primavera, or *all* will be lost. The twelve people are:

1. Samantha Spencer, nineteen, a former Miss Teenage America; enrolled in the drama department of a southern California university

2. Dr. Henry Spencer, forty-three, a marine biologist conducting a research study on Primavera; Nobel Prize recipient

3. Mrs. Renee Spencer, forty-one, housewife and mother

4. Bobby Spencer, thirteen, the youngest Spencer child; mentally retarded

5. Rhonda MacDougall, thirty-three, the owner and director of a multi-million-dollar company, which she built from a $4,000 investment seven years ago

6. Captain Vasily Piotrovich, fifty-nine, the captain of a Russian trawler thought to contain sophisticated spying equipment

7. Wanda Zapotochny, forty-one, first mate and medical officer on the Russian trawler

8. Luis Jimenez, twenty-three, assistant chef at the only hotel on Primavera; the homosexual lover of Karl Sorensen

9. Karl Sorensen, thirty-four, Danish-born maitre d' at the hotel restaurant; Luis Jimenez's roommate and lover

10. Rabbi Sholom Klein, fifty, rabbi of the largest temple in the Northern Hemisphere

11. Arnella Jones, twenty-nine, Jamaican-born hotel maid; an ex-convict

12. Jean-Baptiste Jones, six-week-old son of Arnella Jones

DISCUSSION GUIDELINES

After each of you has identified your choices for the seven survivors, engage in a discussion that considers the following questions:

1. Whom did you select to survive?

2. What were your reasons for the choices?

3. How much agreement and disagreement did you find among your choices?

4. What values do the choices reflect?

5. How do you feel about yourselves in relation to this exercise?

6. Did you use rationalizations to avoid making the decisions in this learning activity (the tsunami is only *expected* to reach Primavera; since Jean-Baptiste weighs only a *few pounds* the helicopter can carry him *and* seven survivors)? What purpose(s) did your rationalizations serve?

6

Staff-Hiring Exercise: A Values Clarification Exercise

DIRECTIONS

You are the director of nursing service of a community hospital in a medium-sized western city. You must immediately replace a very fine intensive care unit staff nurse who died quite suddenly. You must make a choice from among four applicants—Donna, Harriet, Jim, and Beth. From personnel research and interviewing you have learned the following about them:

1. Donna had an exceptional academic record in a baccalaureate nursing program. She is bright and hard working, well liked and well mannered, but she is a very stubborn young woman. She is also a confirmed atheist and does not hide her lack of religious belief. When asked if she intended to meet the spiritual needs of patients and families, she replied that she would do what she believed and that no one had the right to ask her not to. The hospital administrator contends that the hospital owes a duty to the public not to approve a new nurse who holds fanatical ideas about atheism. Donna counters that an employer cannot discriminate against a person on the basis of religion or lack of religion in the United States. She maintains that, if she is qualified, she should be hired.

2. Harriet had an average academic record at a small diploma school of nursing. Her recommendations are just adequate, indicating clearly that some question about her competence remains in the minds of her teachers. When asked how well her previous practice had gone, Harriet replied that she did not finish administering all the care she was supposed to give. The hospital administrator contends that Harriet would be incompetent. Harriet asserts that she is willing and able to learn as she practices.

3. Jim had an exceptional academic record at a large, well-respected, private university. His recommendations were excellent as far as academic preparation was concerned. Jim is well liked by all and well mannered, but he definitely prefers the company of men to that of women. When questioned about this Jim acknowledged that it was true and that he was a homosexual, but he asserted that he had the situation in full control. Jim said that he would not allow any of his homosexual views to influence the performance of his

Source: Adapted with permission of Macmillan Publishing Co., Inc. from COMMUNICATION GAMES by Karen R. Krupar. Copyright ©1973 by The Free Press, a Division of Macmillan Publishing Co., Inc.

role, but, if asked, would acknowledge them. The personnel administrator contends that the hospital has a responsibility to protect its patients from deviants and that exposure to Jim might be a detriment and an injury to patients. Jim contends that his sexual preference is his private life. He has his own circle of friends in a town fifty miles away. He has never been in trouble with the police during four years of undergraduate work and his previous work experiences. He maintains that he is well qualified and that his qualifications should be the basis for his employment.

4. Beth had a sporadic academic record from a large public university. The personnel administrator reports that she is neat, clean, and well dressed. She was a campus radical and took part in several protests, on one occasion spending eighteen days in jail because of her activities. Her record also shows that Beth has strong political leanings toward communism. Upon questioning, Beth admitted her association with certain violent political factions, but she assured the interviewer that she was now ready to settle down. She stressed that she would like to practice on the intensive care unit. The personnel administrator contends that the hospital cannot afford to subject its patients to a Communist. Beth maintains that her political views have nothing to do with her nursing qualifications and that she should be considered for the position.

Which candidate should you select to fill the position?

DISCUSSION GUIDELINES

After each of you has made a choice of a candidate, divide into groups of about five, and discuss the following questions:

1. Did you find the choice difficult? Why or why not?

2. Were any candidates easy to eliminate?

3. What process did you undergo in reaching a decision?

4. What did you learn about yourself and your values from your process and final decision?

7

How Assertive Are You?

This assertiveness tool, although not a validated psychological scale or test, can help you assess your assertiveness. Be honest in your responses.

DIRECTIONS

Next to each statement below, write the number that describes you best, based on the following scale:

0   No or never

1   Somewhat or sometimes

2   About half the time

3   Usually or quite often

4   Almost always or entirely

_____ 1.   When a friend has borrowed my psychiatric nursing textbook and failed to return it as promised, I ask her or him about it.

_____ 2.   I am reluctant to insist that my household mate assumes her or his share of housekeeping tasks.

_____ 3.   When angry, I am likely to use obscenities.

_____ 4.   It disturbs me to have someone observe my clinical work with clients.

_____ 5.   When someone cuts in line ahead of me, I protest directly to the person.

_____ 6.   When another person's smoking disturbs me, I am reluctant to tell the person.

_____ 7.   I am comfortable giving compliments and praising others.

_____ 8.   I find myself saying "I'm sorry" when I don't really mean it.

_____ 9.   I am reluctant to describe myself positively to others.

_____ 10.   I feel uncomfortable making comments or asking questions in class.

_____ 11.   When I differ with a physician I respect, I speak up for my point of view.

_____ 12. If a person criticizes me unfairly I am likely either to hit the person or to leave feeling angry and upset, rather than defend myself verbally.

_____ 13. At a party I am likely to introduce myself and start a conversation with someone I don't know.

_____ 14. I find myself shouting or crying when others don't go along with me.

_____ 15. When my restaurant meal is not prepared or served as it should be, I ask the waiter or waitress to correct the situation.

_____ 16. I find myself speaking for others or making decisions for them.

_____ 17. When I am talking with someone I am able to maintain eye contact with that person.

_____ 18. I am able to refuse a friend a favor if I don't wish to do what my friend asks of me.

_____ 19. When a salesperson waits on someone before me who came to the counter after me, I can call attention to it.

_____ 20. I "fly off the handle."

EXPLANATION OF SCORING

These questions assess assertive versus nonassertive or aggressive behavior. Assertive behavior is self-enhancing, goal-achieving behavior, freely chosen by the person, that honestly expresses that person's feelings. Nonassertive behavior denies the self, inhibits the expression of the person's feelings, allows others to choose for the self, and fails to achieve the individual's desired goals. Aggressive behavior accomplishes the person's own ends, is self-enhancing, and expresses feelings but at the expense of another, thus diminishing the other's freedom of choice and sense of worth.

For some questions in this tool, the assertive end of the scale is 0. For others it is 4. The key below tells you which behaviors are at the ends of the scales.

QUESTION	0 END OF SCALE	4 END OF SCALE
1	nonassertive	assertive
2	assertive	nonassertive
3	assertive	aggressive
4	assertive	nonassertive
5	nonassertive	assertive
6	assertive	nonassertive
7	nonassertive	assertive
8	assertive	nonassertive
9	assertive	nonassertive
10	assertive	nonassertive
11	nonassertive	assertive
12	assertive	aggressive
13	nonassertive	assertive
14	assertive	aggressive
15	nonassertive	assertive
16	assertive	aggressive
17	nonassertive	assertive
18	nonassertive	assertive
19	nonassertive	assertive
20	assertive	aggressive

Add up the number of questions you answered toward the assertive end of the scale. Then get the total you answered toward the other end. To profile your results, draw a line across each column below at the point that represents your score. Shade in the areas from zero to the line you have drawn in each column.

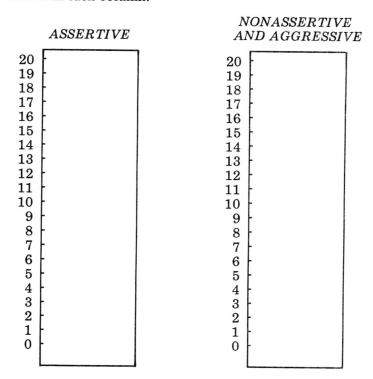

ASSERTIVE

NONASSERTIVE
AND AGGRESSIVE

DISCUSSION GUIDE

After scoring your answers to the twenty questions, divide into small groups to discuss the following:

1. How do nonassertive, assertive, and aggressive behaviors relate to sex roles?

2. Which behaviors are common among nurses? Why?

3. What assertive responses can you formulate for each of the questions in which you scored at the opposite end of the scale?

4. What rights do you believe people should have in their relationships with others?

5. What responsibilities do you believe people should have in their relationships with others?

8

Hurting and Being Hurt

DIRECTIONS

In the space below write twenty sentences in which the word *hurt* is used.

1.

2.

3.

4.

5.

6.

7.

8.

9.

10.

11.

12.

13.

14.

15.

16.

17.

18.

19.

20.

DISCUSSION GUIDELINES

This exercise focuses on the expression of hurt in both the emotional and the physical sense and the ease or difficulty with which you acknowledge being hurt. It may also encourage you to become aware of specific areas of emotional vulnerability. The following questions may be helpful.

1. How often, and in what ways, did you refer to hurt in yourself as opposed to hurt in others?

2. Did you tend to use the word *hurt* in an active or a passive sense?

3. Did you tend to use the word *hurt* in an emotional or a physical sense?

4. Under what circumstances are you hurt?

5. Under what circumstances do you hurt others?

6. How do you reduce emotional hurt within yourself?

9

What Is Your Intimacy Quotient?

This exercise is designed to measure your capacity for intimacy—how well you have fared in (and what you have learned from) your interpersonal relationships from infancy through adulthood. In a general way, it helps measure your sense of security and self-acceptance, which gives you the courage to risk the embarrassment of proffering love or friendship or respect and getting no response. This exercise can provide insight and can alert you to weaknesses that may be reducing your performance in everything from nursing, to meeting and interacting with potential mates, to ordering food in a restaurant.

DIRECTIONS

Read each question carefully. If your response is yes or mostly yes, place a plus (+) on the line preceding the question. If your response is no or mostly no, place a minus (−) on the line. If you honestly can't decide, place a zero (0) on the line; but try to enter as few zeroes as possible. Even if a particular question doesn't apply to you, try to imagine yourself in the situation described and answer accordingly. Don't look for any significance in the number or the frequency of plus or minus answers. Simply be honest when answering the questions.

_____ 1. Do you have more than your share of colds?

_____ 2. Do you believe that emotions have very little to do with physical ills?

_____ 3. Do you often have indigestion?

_____ 4. Do you frequently worry about your health?

_____ 5. Would a nutritionist be appalled by your diet?

_____ 6. Do you usually watch sports rather than participate in them?

_____ 7. Do you often feel depressed or in a bad mood?

Source: Adapted from *Go to Health*, Copyright 1973 by Communications Research Machines, Inc. Used with permission of Delacorte Press.

_____   8. Are you irritable when things go wrong?

_____   9. Were you happier in the past than you are right now?

_____   10. Do you believe it possible that a person's character can be read or one's future foretold by means of astrology, I Ching, tarot cards, or some other means?

_____   11. Do you worry about the future?

_____   12. Do you try to hold in your anger as long as possible and then sometimes explode in a rage?

_____   13. Do people you care about often make you feel jealous?

_____   14. If your intimate partner were unfaithful one time, would you be unable to forgive and forget?

_____   15. Do you have difficulty making important decisions?

_____   16. Would you abandon a goal rather than take risks to reach it?

_____   17. When you go on a vacation, do you take some work along?

_____   18. Do you usually wear clothes that are dark or neutral in color?

_____   19. Do you usually do what you feel like doing, regardless of social pressures or criticism?

_____   20. Does a beautiful speaking voice turn you on?

_____   21. Do you always take an interest in where you are and what's happening around you?

_____   22. Do you find most odors interesting rather than offensive?

_____   23. Do you enjoy trying new and different foods?

_____   24. Do you like to touch and be touched?

_____   25. Are you easily amused?

_____   26. Do you often do things spontaneously or impulsively?

_____   27. Can you sit still through a long committee meeting or lecture without twiddling your thumbs or wriggling in your chair?

_____   28. Can you usually fall asleep and stay asleep without the use of sleeping pills or tranquilizers?

_____   29. Are you a moderate drinker rather than either a heavy drinker or a teetotaler?

_____   30. Do you smoke not at all or very little?

_____   31. Can you put yourself in another person's place and experience their emotions?

_____   32. Are you seriously concerned about social problems even when they don't affect you personally?

_____   33. Do you think most people can be trusted?

_____   34. Can you talk to a celebrity or a stranger as easily as you talk to your neighbors?

_____ 35. Do you get along well with salesclerks, waiters, service-station attendants, and cabdrivers?

_____ 36. Can you easily discuss sex in mixed company without feeling uncomfortable?

_____ 37. Can you express appreciation for a gift or a favor without feeling uneasy?

_____ 38. When you feel affection for someone, can you express it physically as well as verbally?

_____ 39. Do you sometimes feel that you have extrasensory perception?

_____ 40. Do you like yourself?

_____ 41. Do you like others of your own sex?

_____ 42. Do you enjoy an evening alone?

_____ 43. Do you vary your schedule to avoid doing the same things at the same times each day?

_____ 44. Is love more important to you than money or status?

_____ 45. Do you place a higher premium on kindness than on truthfulness?

_____ 46. Do you think it is possible to be too rational?

_____ 47. Have you attended or would like to attend a sensitivity or encounter-group session?

_____ 48. Do you discourage friends from dropping in unannounced?

_____ 49. Would you feel it a sign of weakness to seek help for a sexual problem?

_____ 50. Are you upset when a homosexual seems attracted to you?

_____ 51. Do you have difficulty communicating with someone of the opposite sex?

_____ 52. Do you believe that men who write poetry are less masculine than men who drive trucks?

_____ 53. Do most women prefer men with well-developed muscles to men with well-developed emotions?

_____ 54. Are you generally indifferent to the kind of place in which you live?

_____ 55. Do you consider it a waste of money to buy flowers for yourself or for others?

_____ 56. When you see an art object you like, do you pass it up if the cost would mean cutting back on your food budget?

_____ 57. Do you think it pretentious and extravagant to have an elegant dinner when alone or with members of your immediate family?

_____ 58. Are you often bored?

_____ 59. Do Sundays depress you?

_____ 60. Do you frequently feel nervous?

_____ 61. Do you dislike the work you do to earn a living?

_____ 62. Do you think a carefree hippie life style would have no delights for you?

_____ 63.   Do you watch TV selectively rather than simply to kill time?

_____ 64.   Have you read any good books recently?

_____ 65.   Do you often daydream?

_____ 66.   Do you like to fondle pets?

_____ 67.   Do you like many different forms and styles of art?

_____ 68.   Do you enjoy watching an attractive person of the opposite sex?

_____ 69.   Can you describe how your date or mate looked the last time you went out together?

_____ 70.   Do you find it easy to talk to new acquaintances?

_____ 71.   Do you communicate with others through touch as well as through words?

_____ 72.   Do you enjoy pleasing members of your family?

_____ 73.   Do you avoid joining clubs or organizations?

_____ 74.   Do you worry more about how you present yourself to perspective dates than about how you treat them?

_____ 75.   Are you afraid that if people knew you too well they wouldn't like you?

_____ 76.   Do you fall in love at first sight?

_____ 77.   Do you always fall in love with someone who reminds you of your parent of the opposite sex?

_____ 78.   Do you think love is all you presently need to be happy?

_____ 79.   Do you feel a sense of rejection if a person you love tries to preserve his or her independence?

_____ 80.   Can you accept your loved one's anger and still believe in his or her love?

_____ 81.   Can you express your innermost thoughts and feelings to the person you love?

_____ 82.   Do you talk over disagreements with your partner rather than silently worry about them?

_____ 83.   Can you easily accept the fact that your partner has loved others before you and not worry about how you compare with them?

_____ 84.   Can you accept a partner's disinterest in sex without feeling rejected?

_____ 85.   Can you accept occasional sessions of unsatisfactory sex without blaming yourself or your partner?

_____ 86.   Should unmarried adolescents be denied contraceptives?

_____ 87.   Do you believe that even for adults in private there are some sexual acts that should remain illegal?

_____ 88.   Do you think that hippie communes and Israeli kibbutzim have nothing useful to teach the average American?

_____ 89.   Should a couple put up with an unhappy marriage for the sake of their children?

_____ 90.   Do you think that mate swappers necessarily have unhappy marriages?

_____ 91. Should older men and women be content not to have sex?

_____ 92. Do you believe that pornography contributes to sex crimes?

_____ 93. Is sexual abstinence beneficial to a person's health, strength, wisdom, or character?

_____ 94. Can a truly loving wife or husband sometimes be sexually unreceptive?

_____ 95. Can intercourse during a women's menstrual period be as appealing or as appropriate as at any other time?

_____ 96. Should a woman concentrate on her own sensual pleasure during intercourse rather than pretend enjoyment to increase her partner's pleasure?

_____ 97. Can a man's effort to bring his partner to orgasm reduce his own pleasure?

_____ 98. Should fun and sensual pleasure be the principal goals in sexual relations?

_____ 99. Is pressure to perform well a common cause of sexual incapacity?

_____ 100. Is sexual intercourse for you an uninhibited romp rather than a demonstration of your sexual ability?

EXPLANATION OF SCORING

Questions   1-18, count your minuses   _____

Questions 19-47, count your pluses   _____

Questions 48-62, count your minuses   _____

Questions 63-72, count your pluses   _____

Questions 73-79, count your minuses   _____

Questions 80-85, count your pluses   _____

Questions 86-93, count your minuses   _____

Questions 94-100, count your pluses   _____

Total   _____

Substract from this total half the number of zero answers to obtain your corrected total.

If your corrected total score is under 30, you have a shell like a tortoise and tend to draw your head in at the first sign of psychological danger. Probably life handed you some bad blows when you were too young to fight back, so you've erected strong defenses against the kind of intimacy that could leave you vulnerable to ego injury.

If you scored between 30 and 60, you're about average, which shows you have potential. You've erected some strong defenses, but you've matured enough, and have had enough good experiences, that you're willing to take a few chances with other human beings, confident that you'll survive regardless.

Any score over 60 means you possess the self-confidence and sense of security not only to run the risks of intimacy but to enjoy it. This could be a little discomforting to another person who doesn't have your capacity or potential for close interpersonal relationships, but you're definitely ahead in the game and you can make the right person extremely happy just by being yourself. If your score approaches 100, you're either an intimate superstar or you are worried too much about giving right answers, which puts you back in the under-30 category.

If it is convenient, try taking it with someone you feel intimate with—afterward compare and discuss your answers. It may indicate how compatible you are, socially or sexually. This is one area of interpersonal relationships in which opposites do not necessarily attract. A person of high intimacy capacity can intimidate someone of low capacity who is fearful to respond. But those of similar capacities will tend to make no excessive demands on each other and, for that reason, will find themselves capable of an increasingly intimate and mutually fulfilling relationship.

10

The Ten Commandments

DIRECTIONS

Use the form below to write out as many of the Ten Commandments as you can recall.

THE TEN COMMANDMENTS

Compare your list with the actual commandments below.

1. I am the Lord thy God, which have brought thee out of the land of Egypt, out of the house of bondage. Thou shalt have no other gods before me.

2. Thou shalt not make unto thee any graven image, or any likeness of any thing that is in heaven above, or that is in the earth beneath, or that is in the water under the earth. Thou shalt not bow down thyself to them, nor serve them: for I the Lord thy God am a jealous God, visiting the iniquity of the fathers upon the children unto the third and fourth generation of them that hate me; and shewing mercy unto thousands of them that love me, and keep my commandments.

3. Thou shalt not take the name of the Lord thy God in vain; for the Lord will not hold him guiltless that taketh his name in vain.

4. Remember the sabbath day, to keep it holy. Six days shalt thou labor, and do all thy work. But the seventh day is the sabbath of the Lord thy God: in it thou shalt not do any work, thou, nor thy son, nor thy daughter, thy manservant, nor thy maidservant, nor thy cattle, nor thy sojourner who is within thy gates. For in six days the Lord made heaven and earth, the sea, and all that in them is, and rested the seventh day: wherefore the Lord blessed the sabbath day, and hallowed it.

5. Honor thy father and thy mother: that thy days may be long in the land which the Lord thy God giveth thee.

6. Thou shalt not kill.

7. Thou shalt not commit adultery.

8. Thou shalt not steal.

9. Thou shalt not bear false witness against thy neighbor.

10. Thou shalt not covet thy neighbor's house, thou shalt not covet thy neighbor's wife, nor his manservant, nor his maidservant, nor his ox, nor his ass, nor any thing that is thy neighbor's.

DISCUSSION GUIDELINES

After comparing your list with the actual commandments, discuss the personal significance of your distortions of recall, your omissions, and the order in which you recalled the Ten Commandments.

Now write out ten personal commandments that you would like to be able to follow.

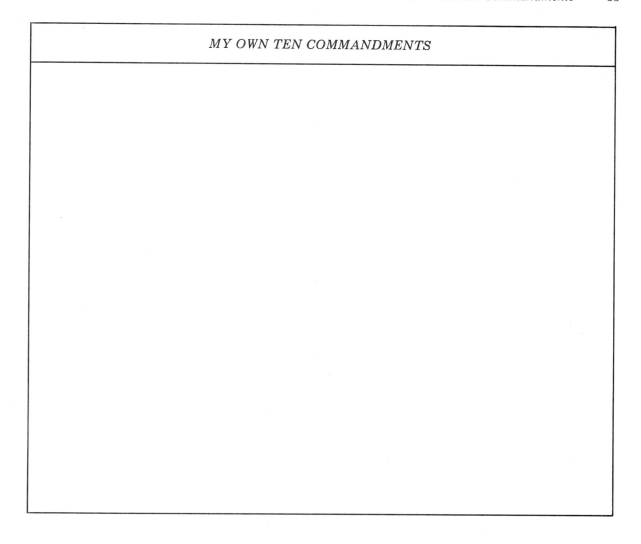

MY OWN TEN COMMANDMENTS

DISCUSSION GUIDELINES

Read your personal commandments aloud to the group and discuss them, considering the following questions:

1. Which commandments are unrealistic? Arbitrary? Coercive? Cliché ridden?

2. What are the relevance and value of each commandment for you?

3. Are cultural myths and shibboleths reflected in your commandments?

4. To what extent may the beliefs and values reflected in your commandments influence your therapeutic interactions with clients?

11

Humanistic Beliefs: Where Do You Stand?

DIRECTIONS

The following statements reflect ideas and beliefs consistent with a humanistic approach to life. Next to each statement below circle "yes" if you agree with the statement and "no" if you disagree with the statement. Be honest in your responses.

1. Natural events have natural causes.   Yes   No

2. The universe is neither for us nor against us; it just doesn't care.   Yes   No

3. Human beings can figure out from experience what's right and wrong.   Yes   No

4. We human beings are responsible, to ourselves and each other, to do what's right.   Yes   No

5. To make it in this life, people need each other.   Yes   No

6. Reason is the most powerful human tool for solving human problems.   Yes   No

7. Scientific method isn't perfect, and it isn't the only way of acquiring knowledge, but it seems to work better than any of the alternatives.   Yes   No

8. Instead of expecting God or the government to take care of human problems, it's better if people get to work on those problems for themselves.   Yes   No

9. Nobody is going to hand you your happiness; you create it yourself.   Yes   No

10. We are not born sinful; we're just born human—born with opportunities, not with burdens of guilt or promises of privilege.   Yes   No

11. What happens to us in this life isn't fixed by the stars and planets or by the gods; very often, it's a consequence of our own choices.   Yes   No

Source: Reproduced by permission of Richard Czarnecki, Editor, 459 Traverse Blvd. Buffalo, NY 14223 *Humanistically Speaking*, March 1981.

12. It's right to be open to learn from other people and to hear their views fairly stated.   Yes   No

13. Individual human freedom of choice is a part of our humanity well worth defending.   Yes   No

14. We human beings are a part of nature—we belong here, and all life is our kin.   Yes   No

15. Human will has the potential to transform the world of human experience.   Yes   No

16. Life is a 'do-it-yourself' job, and there's nobody waiting around to rescue us.   Yes   No

DISCUSSION GUIDELINES

After each of you has responded to the statements discuss the following questions in seminar or small groups.

1. Would you call yourself a humanist? Why? Why not?

2. Was it easier to respond "yes" to some questions than it was to others? If so, can you find a common theme or thread that seems to tie them together?

3. How do your responses fit with each of the following humanistic beliefs?

    a. People have freedom of choice.

    b. People not only can decide their own immediate behavior but can, to some extent, also take charge of their own destiny.

    c. People can refuse the destiny imposed by the accident of time and place of birth and can become capable of making decisions that shape their own destinies.

4. How might your beliefs influence your interactions and effectiveness with clients?

Beware of Sharks:
A Values Clarification Exercise

The following structured exercise, having to do with values clarification, will help you to increase your self-awareness.

DIRECTIONS

Read the story and follow the instructions.

The Story

Five people took a cruise. The five people were: A, B, C, D, and E. A and B were in love and planned to marry the next week. A storm came up and the boat was tossed and battered. It hit a rock and capsized between two islands. A, C, and D managed to swim to one island; B and E made it to the other.

Source: Virgil Parsons and Nancy Sanford, *Interpersonal Interaction in Nursing: Basic Concepts in Nurse-Patient Communication*, pp. 33-35, Copyright © 1979 by Addison-Wesley Publishing Company, Menlo Park, CA.

A and B were separated, and A was heartbroken. A wanted to get to B as soon as possible. But there was a problem. Sharks! (Shades of *Jaws*.) The water between the islands was full of them. A was determined to reach B some way. A loved B and felt a need to be together.

A got an idea: C or D could help build a raft and sail across to B. A went to C and asked for help. C studied the problem and finally said, "The odds are against it. If we did build a raft, the materials wouldn't hold up. Besides it's so windy, and the ocean is so rough, that it just isn't feasible. No, I'm sorry, but it's too risky." So A went to D. D looked A in the eye, and said, "Yes. For a price." A was stunned, said, "Never!" and ran away.

Finally it became unbearable. A just could not live without B any longer and so gave in to D. They built a raft and somehow managed to reach the other island.

A was very happy and ran straight to B. But B pushed A away and said, "I know how you got over here. I don't want anything to do with you." A dissolved in tears, crying, "I only did it for you. I wanted to be with you. Can't you understand that?" But B was steadfast. Meanwhile, E, overhearing all this, thought B was a jerk. E went to A and said, "Anyone who would go through all that for the love of another person must be pretty special. If you will have me A, I'd be glad to marry you."

Okay, you have read the story. Now, list the characters in the order you prefer them. In other words, rate the people in order, from the person you respect most to the one you respect least.

1.   2.   3.   4.   5.

Two different interpretations of what each character symbolizes appear below.

CHARACTER	INTERPRETATION #1	INTERPRETATION #2
A	love	sex
B	morals	morality
C	education	business-like
D	sex	power
E	family	security

Using whichever interpretation seems more logical to you, list your own hierarchy of values, as indicated by your above choices.

1.

2.

3.

4.

5.

DISCUSSION GUIDELINES

The reliability of the interpretations will not be argued here. For the present, accept them as valid. Divide into groups of five to compare your hierarchy of values with those of the others in your group, considering these questions:

1. What are the major differences?

2. What are the major similarities?

3. Did your hierarchy surprise you?

4. If you had the opportunity would you reorder the words or substitute other words?

5. How did this exercise increase your self-awareness?

13

Who's In Charge: Your Parent, Adult, or Child?

This learning activity is based on transactional analysis theory.* Three different ego states, Parent, Adult, and Child, are represented in three scales of fifteen items each.

DIRECTIONS

Look at the three sets of statements below. If you agree more than you disagree with a statement, mark a plus (+) beside it. If you disagree more than you agree, mark a minus (−). Be sure to place either a plus or a minus to the left of each number.

The Parent Scale

( ) 1. People today just don't have enough courage to stand up for what is right.

( ) 2. The effective psychiatric nurse is a strong, tough-minded sort of person.

( ) 3. Severe punishment is justified because it stops people from doing wrong.

( ) 4. If divorces were not so easy to obtain, marriages would be taken more seriously.

( ) 5. Patients are better off if they accept what the hospital staff tells them rather than adopt a questioning approach.

( ) 6. I tend to make statements that begin with "You should," "They ought," "It's never," etc.

( ) 7. Suicide is wrong.

( ) 8. I tend to want to run things or take charge.

( ) 9. Patients don't have enough respect for nurses and doctors.

( ) 10. People who are too submissive, ingratiating, or vacillating anger or disgust me.

( ) 11. Nurses should be more dedicated to certain fundamental truths about morals, right and wrong, human nature, and so on.

*See Eric Berne, *Transactional Analysis in Psychotherapy* (New York: Grove Press, 1961).

( ) 12.   It's unfortunate, but no matter how hard you try, you can't change human nature.

( ) 13.   Minority groups get all the breaks.

( ) 14.   I believe that hospital wards function better when the head nurse enforces rules strictly.

( ) 15.   I tend to blame others for what happens more than I would like to.

The Adult Scale

( ) 1.   Patients to whom I've given nursing care would say I'm decisive, yet they don't seem reluctant to disagree with me.

( ) 2.   Most mistakes that people make result from misunderstanding rather than carelessness.

( ) 3.   I seldom if ever blush.

( ) 4.   Before starting some action I tend to gather facts and form a plan.

( ) 5.   I find opinions and ideas that differ from my own interesting.

( ) 6.   When I was a child, my parents encouraged me to express my views.

( ) 7.   I don't usually feel bored, impatient, or lonely.

( ) 8.   When it seems appropriate I can express my emotions.

( ) 9.   I have attended, or would like to attend, a self-awareness or growth group.

( ) 10.   Patients seem to turn to me for advice, counsel, etc., more than they turn to many nurses.

( ) 11.   I find that I'm more able than most people to present a calm exterior even though I am churning inside.

( ) 12.   It is possible to be honest and truthful with others.

( ) 13.   I seem to have little need to dominate patients, but I also seldom, if ever, feel dominated by them.

( ) 14.   People are capable of sustained self-direction and control.

( ) 15.   I seem to be more comfortable than many people I know with a long period of silence.

The Child Scale

( ) 1.   Humor seems to be a good way to lessen the tension in situations that are too serious.

( ) 2.   I find myself becoming upset when I don't get my own way.

( ) 3.   Perhaps more so than others, I'm concerned when patients display their negative emotions such as anger, boredom, etc.

( ) 4.   Most important life decisions are made on the basis of feelings rather than logic.

( ) 5.   I'm overconcerned about the approval of others.

( ) 6. If a psychiatrist or someone with higher authority than I have assumes the responsibility for a "tough" decision that imposes a considerable hardship on some people, I'll help carry it out.

( ) 7. I seem to cry more than most people do.

( ) 8. Sometimes I catch myself laughing too loudly or talking too loudly.

( ) 9. I feel more comfortable in "structured" situations.

( ) 10. Persons in positions of higher authority often belittle their subordinates.

( ) 11. I don't understand why, but there are times when I seem to get the "short end of the stick."

( ) 12. Driving very fast is fun.

( ) 13. There are times when I've told patients or their families "I don't make the rules, I just follow them."

( ) 14. I find sticking to a diet or quitting smoking difficult.

( ) 15. Expressions such as "Gosh," "Gee," "Golly," "Wow," are quite common in my vocabulary.

EXPLANATION OF SCORING

Each scale is scored separately. Each item answered by a plus is given a raw score of 1. Minus answers are given 0. Scores for each scale can thus range from a high of 15 to a low of 0. To profile your results, add the totals for each scale and draw a line across each column below at the point that represents your score. Shade in the area between zero and the line you have drawn in each column.

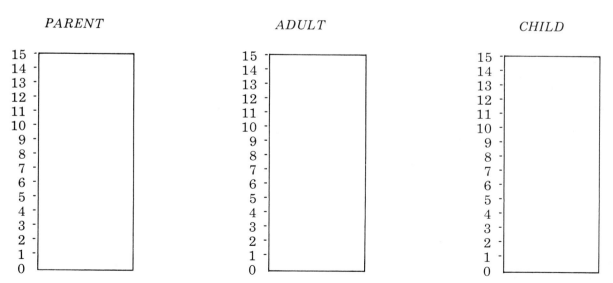

Parent score: This represents the extent to which your behavior resembles that of a parent. This ego state is characterized by automatic use of words such as "cute," "sonny," "ought," "should," "must," "always," "disgusting," "naughty," etc. The Parent is "never wrong."

Adult score: This represents the extent to which your behavior is a function of logical processing of facts offered by the here-and-now environment. This ego state also engages in probability estimating. The Adult says, "I will."

Child score: This represents the extent to which your behavior resembles that of children. In this ego state, oaths, exclamations, name calling, and the use of such words as "gee," "I'll try," and "maybe" are typical.

Your highest raw score indicates the ego state you use most. The greater the difference between this score and your next highest score, the more dominant the ego state. The lesser the difference the more likely it is that you switch back and forth between the two ego states.

It is desirable that the Adult ego state be dominant. Most people want to increase their Adult and decrease their Parent. The Child ego state is of less concern, unless it is either too high or too low. Some typical problem profiles are:

· High Parent, low Adult, low Child (the Archie Bunker type)

· Low Parent, low Adult, high Child (Edith Bunker, Archie's wife)

DISCUSSION GUIDELINES

After you have each arrived at your total scores for each ego state, discuss the ego states by name, considering these questions:

1. What in your life experience might have led to the dominance of one ego state over another? To similarity in strength of two ego states?

2. Would you have been able to predict your ego state scores?

3. How might your ego states influence your interactions and effectiveness with psychiatric clients?

14

The Valois
Sexual Attitudes Questionnaire

This exercise is designed for you to respond to a number of statements dealing with human sexuality in our culture and for you to analyze your sexual attitudes on a liberal conservative or accepting/nonaccepting continuum.

DIRECTIONS

Read each statement carefully and indicate your reaction to each statement by placing in the space provided at the left of each question: SA=Strongly Agree, A=Agree, D=Disagree, or SD=Strongly Disagree.

Response

_____ 1. Homosexuals should be put in a place where the rest of society does not have to put up with them.

_____ 2. Masturbation by a married person is a sign of poor marital adjustment.

_____ 3. Mouth-genital contact can provide a higher degree of effective erotic stimulation than can sexual intercourse.

_____ 4. Sex education should not be taught in the schools.

_____ 5. The practice of birth control is worthwhile.

_____ 6. Premarital intercourse between consenting adults is acceptable.

_____ 7. College marriages are usually doomed to failure.

_____ 8. Venereal disease is only contracted by lower socioeconomic people.

_____ 9. Rape is an easy crime to commit and never be convicted of this crime.

Source: Reprinted by permission from Stafford Cox et al., *Wellness R.S.V.P.*, Menlo Park, CA: The Benjamin/Cummings Publishing Company, 1981, pp. 52-54.

_____ 10. Abortion should be prohibited under all circumstances.

_____ 11. Pornography has a detrimental impact upon moral character and therefore is related to crimes of a sexual nature.

_____ 12. Living together is only practiced by white middle-class youth.

_____ 13. Sexual intercourse is a kind of communication.

_____ 14. Homosexuals should not be employed in occupations where they might serve as role models.

_____ 15. Masturbation is accepted when the objective is simply the attainment of sensory enjoyment.

_____ 16. Mouth-genital contact should be regarded as an acceptable form of erotic play.

_____ 17. Sex education should be as common a school subject as math or English.

_____ 18. Birth control is as much a man's responsibility as a woman's responsibility.

_____ 19. Sexual intercourse should occur only between married partners.

_____ 20. College marriages are no different from any other marriages.

_____ 21. Masturbation is generally unhealthy.

_____ 22. Preserving the physical health of the mother should be the only basis for abortion.

_____ 23. Communication barriers are the key factors causing sexual problems.

_____ 24. Homosexuality should be regarded as an illness.

_____ 25. Relieving tension by masturbation is a healthy practice.

_____ 26. Women should be as willing as men to participate in mouth-genital sex play.

_____ 27. Too much fuss is made over sex education.

_____ 28. The practice of birth control leads to increased sexual activity.

_____ 29. Women should experience sexual intercourse prior to marriage.

_____ 30. It takes a mature couple to make a college marriage work.

_____ 31. Venereal disease does not exist among upper and middle class people.

_____ 32. The ultimate goal of rape is sexual satisfaction.

_____ 33. Abortion is murder.

_____ 34. Pornography is not harmful to young children and there is no need to be concerned about their coming in contact with it.

_____ 35. Living together often indicates a strong sexual need for each partner.

_____ 36. The basis of sexual communication is touching.

_____ 37. Homosexuality repulses me.

_____ 38. Mouth-genital contact repulses me.

_____ 39. Sex education at the college level serves no purpose.

_____ 40. Birth control pills should be available at a college health service.

——— 41. Men should experience sexual intercourse prior to marriage.

——— 42. College marriages add but one more problem to an already frustrating time of life.

——— 43. Rape usually occurs within a mile of the victim's home.

——— 44. Abortion should be permitted whenever desired by the mother.

——— 45. Masturbation should be encouraged under certain conditions.

——— 46. Homosexuality is all right between two consenting adults.

EXPLANATION OF SCORING

After responding to these statements compare your results with friends, classmates, and the person you are in a relationship with (if applicable). Discussion of these statements will help make clear that we all differ in our sexual values and that we bring these differences into a relationship. It will be helpful to group your responses by topic as follows:

Sexual stereotypes: Questions 4, 8, 9, 11, 17, 27, 31, 32, 34, 39, and 43. These items refer to sexual items that tend to be stereotypical in nature and exist prior to formal sex education at the college level.

Masturbation: Questions 2, 15, 21, 25, and 45 refer to the sexual behavior of masturbation.

Premarital intercourse: Questions 6, 12, 19, 29, 35, and 41 deal with premarital intercourse in our society.

Homosexuality: Questions 1, 14, 24, 37, and 46 indicate attitudes toward the sexual orientation of homosexuality.

Sexual communication: Questions 13, 23, and 36 deal with the process of sexual communication in a sexual situation and within a relationship.

College marriages: Questions 7, 20, 30, and 42 refer to getting married while still in college or academic pursuit.

Abortion: Questions 10, 22, 33, and 44 address the topic of abortion in our culture.

Oral-genital sex: Questions 3, 16, 26, and 38 explore attitudes toward the practice of mouth-genital sex in our society.

Birth control: Questions 5, 18, 28, and 40 refer to the practice of birth control and responsibility for it.

15

The Great Blizzard: How Leadership Emerges

An unrelenting blizzard of enormous proportions has virtually paralyzed a large eastern city located on one of the Great Lakes. "White-outs" caused by forty-mile-per-hour howling winds, gusting to fifty-five, have stranded anyone unfortunate enough to be away from home. Roads and highways are impassable, with drifts rising to ten feet. Smaller buildings and houses are blocked by the high drifts and by cars completely covered with snow.

The mayor and county executive have just declared a state of emergency. Meteorologists with the National Weather Service predict an unprecedented snowfall, with high winds continuing for the next seventy-two to ninety-six hours. The outdoor temperature is 10° F. However, the high winds have brought the chill factor to −22° F. Overnight the temperature is expected to reach 0° F. with a −35° F. wind chill factor. The metropolitan Department of Streets and Highways has declared that cleanup and removal efforts cannot even begin until the snow and winds subside.

Thirty-one people find themselves stranded in a popular restaurant and bar. Some are women and children who were out shopping and left their stranded automobiles to seek shelter from the cold and wind. Others are workers who had set out to reach their suburban homes. A few are patrons. Because there was a large political fund-raising party at the restaurant the evening before and several delivery trucks failed to arrive earlier that afternoon, many of the restaurant's food stores are depleted. Although there is a large supply of liquor, there is sufficient food for thirty-one people for only two days. Newscasters have been warning of the possibility of food, gas, electricity, and water shortages or malfunctions. Among the thirty-one marooned persons are the following eight:

Sister Mary Marcia Sutter, twenty-nine, a Catholic nun, the elected head of Religious for Ecumenical Freedom, an outspoken group of nuns and priests opposed to the conservative views of the bishop of the diocese.

Jerry ("The Fox") Rosso, forty-five, an underworld don and the owner of the Riviera, the restaurant and bar hosting the stranded travelers.

Irene Ostrander, thirty-six, chief administrator of an 800-bed general hospital and an ambitious community leader.

Dr. C. Elizabeth Byrd, forty, a clinical psychologist in private practice and a crisis consultant to community caretaker groups such as the state police and local fire department.

Jean-Jacques Krause, twenty-five, a former Olympic downhill ski racer, on his way to Blue Mountain to serve as director of the ski school and manager of Quest, its outdoor survival training program.

Louie Boles, forty-seven, a former air force career officer, now the public relations man for a United States senator.

Shirley Monroe, fifty, an attorney and a candidate for judge of the family court.

Paul Wolchyk, thirty-seven, the owner of a string of shoe,stores and a small business management consultant.

DIRECTIONS

In groups of about five, take up to thirty minutes to decide which of these eight persons would emerge in a leadership role. How would the leadership come about? Why?

DISCUSSION GUIDELINES

1. What conditions in the story influenced the decisions your group made?

2. Identify the values that influenced you to select one person over another.

3. Did you place greater importance on maintaining good relationships among the stranded persons or on accomplishing the task of survival?

16

Self-Actualization Inventory

The purpose of this exercise is to make you aware of the characteristics of self-actualization and to help you find out whether you are a self-actualizing person, that is, a person who is fulfilling his or her potentials, including esthetic, creative, and spirtual potentials.

DIRECTIONS

Circle the number in the column on the right side that you feel honestly describes how you feel or behave.

CHARACTERISTICS	FREQUENCY			
	VERY OFTEN	OFTEN	SOME-TIMES	NEVER
1. Judge others accurately	5	3	1	0
2. Detect falseness in others	5	3	1	0
3. Tolerate uncertainty	5	3	1	0
4. Accept your good and bad aspects	5	3	1	0
5. Accept others even though you disagree with them	5	3	1	0
6. Get creative ideas	5	3	1	0
7. Enjoy doing unplanned and unrehearsed things	15	10	4	0
8. Involved with problems of others	10	7	3	0

Source: From Walter D. Sorochan, *Personal Health Appraisal*, Copyright 1976. John Wiley & Sons, Inc. Reprinted by permission.

CHARACTERISTICS	FREQUENCY			
	VERY OFTEN	OFTEN	SOME-TIMES	NEVER
9. Able to be alone (by yourself)	10	7	3	0
10. Able to be honest when with strangers	5	3	1	0
11. Resist local customs and traditions	15	10	4	0
12. Have your friends support you before making decisions	5	3	1	0
13. Able to make decisions	5	3	1	0
14. Get a lot of enjoyment from playing or socializing with others	5	3	1	0
15. Appreciate seeing a play or concert	5	3	1	0
16. Feel inspired after hearing or seeing outstanding artists/persons perform	5	3	1	0
17. Have empathy for how another person feels	5	3	1	0
18. Help others to grow and become better persons	5	3	1	0
19. Have deep and meaningful relationships with a few friends	5	3	1	0
20. Feel that a person should be hired on ability and competence	5	3	1	0
21. Do work that you enjoy	10	7	3	0
22. Feel that your work is important	5	3	1	0
23. Laugh at yourself	10	7	3	0
24. Look forward to new experiences	10	7	3	0
25. Enjoy peak and unusual experiences	15	12	4	0
26. Believe that honesty is the best policy	5	3	1	0
27. Believe that one should always tell the truth	5	3	1	0
28. Have dedication to life or social purpose	10	7	3	0
TOTAL _____				

EXPLANATION OF SCORING

Add the numbers you circled. This is your self-actualization score. Classify your score in the appropriate score range.

SCORE RANGE	*CURRENT POTENTIAL FOR SELF-ACTUALIZATION*
150-200	High self-actualization
112-149	Moderate self-actualization
80-111	Approaching self-actualization
0-79	Below average self-actualization

17

Social Support Inventory

The following questions are designed to help you identify your social supports. After completing the inventory, you should be able to determine if you have adequate support. The inventory will also help you identify the types of support you might need and who in your life might provide this support.

OUTSIDE YOUR WORK ENVIRONMENT

1. Who in your life provides you with support by meeting your emotional needs (giving love, listening to your concerns, offering a shoulder to cry on, giving praise)?

2. Do you feel supported by your relatives?

3. Are your close personal friends nurturing, understanding, *and* available?

4. Are there people who meet your informational needs (give moral, ethical, or spiritual advice, for example, a religious leader, teacher, therapist, guru; give financial or legal advice; give health care advice)?

5. Are there people who meet your service needs (child care, house/apartment sitting, transportation, repair people you trust)?

6. Do you know your neighbors and feel that you're a part of your neighborhood?

7. Do you belong to social clubs/organizations in your community (church, civic groups, PTA)?

8. Do you support political, ecological, or social groups that endorse your beliefs?

9. How frequently do you get together with friends by phone or for visits?

10. Are there people whom you care about and enjoy being with but whom you haven't seen recently? If so, what's stopping you from getting together with them?

Source: Adapted from: Smythe EEM: *Surviving Nursing* (Addison-Wesley, 1984), pp. 230–231.

IN YOUR WORK ENVIRONMENT

1. Are there co-workers with whom you can talk about job and/or personal concerns?

2. Are co-workers willing to provide help with patient care?

3. Are there nursing experts in your work setting who provide needed expertise and advice (in-service personnel, supervisors, experienced co-workers)? Are they available?

4. Is your supervisor emotionally supportive and understanding? Does your supervisor seem competent? Is your supervisor available?

5. Are there people at work whose criticism and feedback you value and find useful?

6. Do co-workers encourage your professional advancement/growth?

7. Are there adequate ancillary services (pharmacy, transportation, social service) and equipment in your job?

8. Are you active in your professional organizations?

9. Are there organized staff group meetings where you work (regular nursing care plan meetings, staff meetings, support groups, team meetings, interdisciplinary meetings)?

10. Do you belong to any committees at your place of work?

11. Do you seek out educational opportunities for furthering your professional growth?

DISCUSSION GUIDELINES

In a small group, discuss the following:

1. Who are the persons or groups who provide your best source(s) of support?
2. Which components of your support system need to be enhanced?
3. How can you enhance or enlarge your support system? Give specifics.
4. What do you do to encourage others to support you?
5. What do you do that discourages others from supporting you?

18

Self-Assessment Tool

Therapeutic use of self as a psychiatric nurse requires that you know yourself and your own personal needs before trying to help another person. Your unrecognized and unmet needs may interfere with your ability to be helpful.

DIRECTIONS

On the list below, rank the depth of your own personal needs, according to the following scale:

1 Minimal   4 Quite a bit

2 Little   5 Very high

3 Some

Complete this task individually, and engage in introspection.

____ 1. Like	____ 12. Take care of
____ 2. Be liked	____ 13. Be taken care of
____ 3. Control	____ 14. Succeed
____ 4. Be controlled	____ 15. Be wanted
____ 5. Love	____ 16. Be aggressive
____ 6. Be loved	____ 17. Judge
____ 7. Be stubborn	____ 18. Be judged
____ 8. Be accepted	____ 19. Seek approval
____ 9. Be pleasant	____ 20. Be included
____ 10. Rescue	
____ 11. Be rescued	

DISCUSSION GUIDELINES

With a peer, discuss your identification of personal needs, their depth, the life experiences that may have influenced these needs, the behaviors you generally use to see that your needs are met, and the possible effects of such needs on your interactions with clients and colleagues.

19

Wellness Inventory

Set aside time for yourself to complete this inventory, and find a quiet place where you will not be disturbed while responding to the statements. Using the 3 headings of the columns on the left side of each page as a guide, record your score in one of the blanks alongside each statement.

    2 = Yes, always, or usually

    1 = Sometimes, maybe

    0 = No, rarely

Select the one which best indicates how true the statement is for you *at this time*.

After you have responded to all the appropriate statements in each section, compute an average score from that section, and transfer that number to the Wellness Inventory Wheel on the last page of the questionnaire. When you have colored in the appropriate area between each spoke, you will have a clear presentation of the way in which you balance the many dimensions of your life. The information can be valuable to you to facilitate your growth in the areas of your choosing.

You will find some of the statements are really two in one. This was done to show an important relationship. If only one of them is true for you, check the middle column, giving yourself one point.

Many of the statements have further elaboration in the footnotes, to make their points clearer to you. If a statement indicates it has a footnote, please refer to the footnote before responding.

This questionnaire was designed to educate rather than test. Each statement describes what is believed to be a wellness attribute. The higher your score, the more of these attributes you believe to be true for yourself. It has been necessary to word some of the statements in the negative, i.e., "I don't smoke." If you do smoke, you would give yourself a lower score by saying, in effect, "no, it's not true that I don't smoke." See sample question 3 below. There are no trick questions to test your honesty or consistency—the higher the score, the greater you believe your wellness to be. All statements are worded so that you can tell what the more desirable answer is. This places full responsibility on you to answer each statement as honestly

Source: Abridged from the "Wellness Index," contained in *Wellness Workbook* by R.S. Ryan and J.W. Travis, Ten Speed Press, Berkeley, Ca., 1981. For further information contact Wellness Associates, 42 Miller Avenue, Mill Valley, Ca 94941.

as possible. Remember, it's not your score, but what you learn about yourself, that counts the most with this questionnaire.

EXAMPLE:

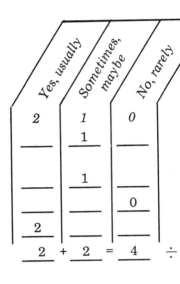

1. I am an adventurous thinker, and I am willing to consider new ideas in consciousness, education and society.

2. I have no expectations, yet look to the future optimistically.

3. I do not smoke.

4. I love long, hot baths.
   average score for this section
   Transfer to Wellness Inventory Wheel at end of activity.

*SECTION 1—WELLNESS, SELF RESPONSIBILITY
AND LOVE*

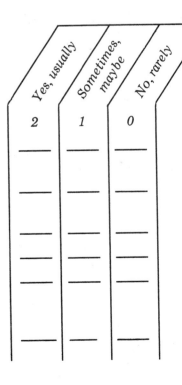

1. How I live my life is an important factor in determining my state of health.

2. I take an active interest in community, national and world events.

3. I feel financially secure.

4. I don't waste energy and materials at home or at work.

5. I take measures to protect my living area from fire and safety hazards (such as improper sized fuses and storage of volatile chemicals).

6. I use dental floss and a soft toothbrush, and have been instructed in their proper use.*

Section 1. 6. Regular flossing and using a good, soft toothbrush with rounded tip bristles prevent the premature loss of teeth in your 40s and 50s. Be sure to learn the proper techniques of use from a dental hygienist or dentist.

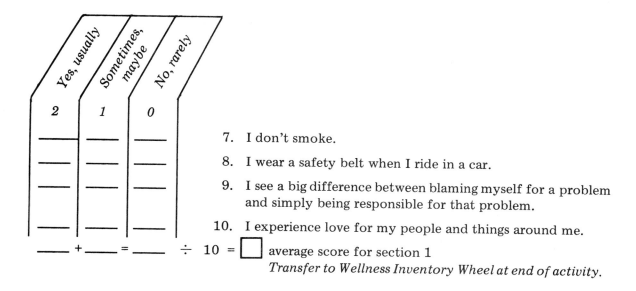

7. I don't smoke.

8. I wear a safety belt when I ride in a car.

9. I see a big difference between blaming myself for a problem and simply being responsible for that problem.

10. I experience love for my people and things around me.

_____ + _____ = _____ ÷ 10 = ☐ average score for section 1

Transfer to Wellness Inventory Wheel at end of activity.

SECTION 2—WELLNESS AND BREATHING

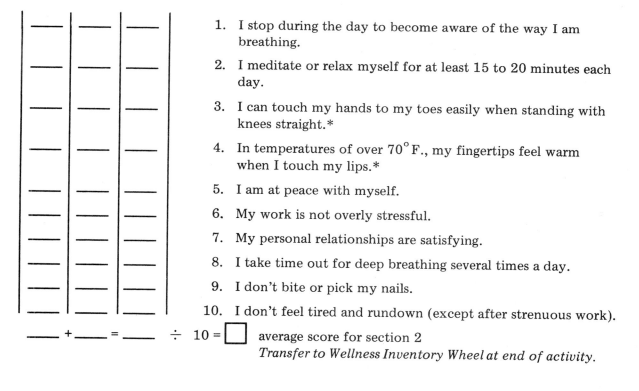

1. I stop during the day to become aware of the way I am breathing.

2. I meditate or relax myself for at least 15 to 20 minutes each day.

3. I can touch my hands to my toes easily when standing with knees straight.*

4. In temperatures of over 70°F., my fingertips feel warm when I touch my lips.*

5. I am at peace with myself.

6. My work is not overly stressful.

7. My personal relationships are satisfying.

8. I take time out for deep breathing several times a day.

9. I don't bite or pick my nails.

10. I don't feel tired and rundown (except after strenuous work).

_____ + _____ = _____ ÷ 10 = ☐ average score for section 2

Transfer to Wellness Inventory Wheel at end of activity.

Section 2. 3. A lack of spinal flexibility is another sympton of chronic muscle tension. 4. When finger temperatures are below 85°F (feel cool to the touch—lips are a good temperature to compare them with) and you are in a relatively warm environment (70°F or more), there is a high likelihood that anxiety is present or your mind is being overly active. Blood circulation to, and hence temperature of, the periphery of your body is reduced by the constriction of small arteries—another response of the sympathetic nervous system to anxiety. Many "cold handers" are completely unaware of this stress sign unless they consciously check hand temperature several times daily.

SECTION—WELLNESS AND SENSING

Yes, usually 2	Sometimes, maybe 1	No, rarely 0	
____	____	____	1. I take long walks, hikes, and/or outings to actively explore my surroundings.
____	____	____	2. I give myself presents, treats, or nurture myself in other ways.
____	____	____	3. I enjoy getting backrubs or massages.
____	____	____	4. I enjoy touching and hugging other people.*
____	____	____	5. I enjoy being touched and hugged by others.*
____	____	____	6. At times I like to be alone.
____	____	____	7. I like getting compliments and recognition from other people.
____	____	____	8. It is easy for me to give other people sincere compliments and recognition.
____	____	____	9. My place of work has largely natural lighting or full-spectrum lighting.*
____	____	____	10. I avoid extremely noisy areas (or wear protective earplugs).*

____ + ____ = ____ ÷ 10 = ☐ average score for section 3
Transfer to Wellness Inventory Wheel at end of activity.

SECTION 4—WELLNESS AND EATING

___	___	___	1. I am aware of the difference between refined carbohydrates (white flour, sugar, etc.) and complex (natural) carbohydrates.**

*Section 3. 4, 5. Touch is one of the most unrecognized human needs for sensory input. "Plastic" or insincere touching or hugging is probably worse than none at all, however.
9. Glass windows and most artificial lighting severely limit the amount of "near" ultraviolet light reaching our eyes. Recent evidence shows a strong link between one's health and the amount of full spectrum light (natural or unfiltered sunlight and certain types of specially designed artificial lamps) which enters our eyes. Eyeglasses can be obtained with a special type of plastic lens which admits the important "near" ultraviolet light.
10. Very loud noises which leave your ears ringing can cause permanent hearing loss which accumulates with years and is usually not noticeable until one reaches 40 or 50. Small cushioned ear plugs (not the type designed for swimmers), wax ear plugs and acoustic ear muffs (which look like stereo headphones without wires) can often be purchased in sporting goods stores and should be worn in noise environments (around power tools, hammers used in confined spaces, loud music, heavy equipment, etc.).

**Section 4. 1. Refined carbohydrates (sugar, white flour, white rice, and alcohol) have only calories and no minerals or vitamins. They are usually rapidly absorbed by the body, quickly burned, and leave a letdown feeling soon afterwards. Natural carbohydrates (fruits, vegetables, whole grains, legumes) contain a good selection of minerals and vitamins. They require time for digestion and hence provide a slower, steadier source of energy over a longer period of time.

	Yes, usually 2	Sometimes, maybe 1	No, rarely 0
2. I am satisfied with my diet.	——	——	——
3. I have fewer than five alcoholic beverages per week and fewer than three cups of coffee or tea per day (except for herbal teas).*	——	——	——
4. I don't take medications, including prescription drugs.	——	——	——
5. I drink fewer than five soft drinks per week.*	——	——	——
6. I add little or no salt to my food.*	——	——	——
7. I read the labels for the ingredients of the foods I buy.	——	——	——
8. I eat at least two raw fruits or vegetables each day.	——	——	——
9. I have a good appetite and maintain a weight within 15% of my ideal weight.	——	——	——
10. I know and feel the difference between "stomach hunger" and "mouth hunger."*	——	——	——

—— + —— = —— ÷ 10 = ☐ average score for section 4
Transfer to Wellness Inventory Wheel at end of activity.

SECTION 5—WELLNESS AND MOVING

——	——	——	1. I climb stairs rather than ride elevators.**
——	——	——	2. My daily activities include moderate physical effort (such as rearing young children, gardening, scrubbing floors, or work which involves being on my feet, etc.).

*Section 4. 3. Coffee and tea (other than herbal teas) contain stimulants which, if abused, do not allow your body to function normally.
5. Soft drinks are high in refined sugar which provides only "empty" calories and usually replace foods which have more nutritional value. Artificially sweetened soft drinks consumed in excess may have long-range consequences as yet not known. (Both types of soft drinks contain caffeine or other stimulants.)
6. Salting foods during cooking draws many vitamins out of the food and into the water which is usually discarded. Heavy salting of foods at the table may cause a strain on the kidneys and result in high blood pressure.
10. "Stomach hunger" is felt in the stomach and is a signal from the body that its cells need nutrients. "Mouth hunger" is experienced in the oral cavity as a desire to chew or suck something and is often a substitute craving for another more basic need such as being touched or acknowledged by self or others.

**Section 5. 1. If a long elevator ride is necessary, try getting off five flights below your destination and walking the rest of the way. You may need to apply pressure to building managers to keep stair doors unlocked.

Yes, usually 2	Sometimes, maybe 1	No, rarely 0	
___	___	___	3. My daily activities include vigorous physical effort (such as heavy construction work, farming, moving heavy objects by hand, etc.).
___	___	___	4. I run at least one mile five times a week (or equivalent aerobic exercise).*
___	___	___	5. I run at least three miles four times a week or equivalent (if this statement is true, mark the item above true as well).
___	___	___	6. I do some form of stretching/limbering exercise for 10 to 20 minutes at least three times per week.*
___	___	___	7. I do yoga or some form of stretching exercise for 15 to 20 minutes at least four times a week (if this statement is true, mark the statement above true as well).
___	___	___	8. I enjoy exploring new and effective ways of caring for myself through movement of my body.
___	___	___	9. I enjoy stretching, moving, and exerting my body.
___	___	___	10. I am aware of and respond to messages from my body about its needs for movement.

___ + ___ = ___ ÷ 10 = ☐ average score for section 5
Transfer to Wellness Inventory Wheel at end of activity.

SECTION 6—WELLNESS AND FEELING

2	1	0	
___	___	___	1. I allow myself to experience a full range of emotions— anger, fear, sadness, and joy—and find constructive ways to express them.**
___	___	___	2. I am able to say "no" to people without feeling guilty.
___	___	___	3. It is easy for me to laugh.

*Section 5. 4. Vigorous aerobic exercise (such as running) must keep the heart rate at approximately 120-150 beats per minute for 12 to 20 minutes to produce the "training effect." Less vigorous aerobic exercise (lower heart rate) must be maintained for much longer periods to produce the same benefit The "training effect" is necessary to prepare the heart for meeting extra strain.
6. Such exercise prevents stiffness of joints and musculo-skeletal degeneration. It also promotes a greater feeling of well-being.

**Section 6. 1. Basic emotions, if repressed, often cause anxiety, depression, irrational behavior or physical disease. People can relearn to feel and express their emotions with a resulting improvement in their well-being. Finding constructive ways to express these emotions (so that all parties concerned feel better) leads to more satisfying relationships and problem solving. Some people, however, exaggerate emotions to control and manipulate others; this can be detrimental to their well-being.

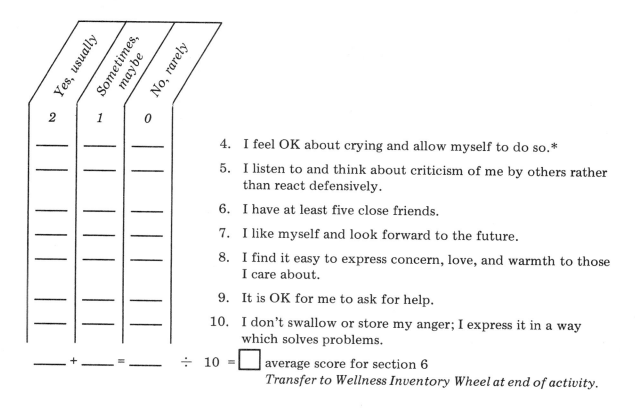

Yes, usually — 2
Sometimes, maybe — 1
No, rarely — 0

4. I feel OK about crying and allow myself to do so.*

5. I listen to and think about criticism of me by others rather than react defensively.

6. I have at least five close friends.

7. I like myself and look forward to the future.

8. I find it easy to express concern, love, and warmth to those I care about.

9. It is OK for me to ask for help.

10. I don't swallow or store my anger; I express it in a way which solves problems.

_____ + _____ = _____ ÷ 10 = ☐ average score for section 6
Transfer to Wellness Inventory Wheel at end of activity.

SECTION 7—WELLNESS AND THINKING

1. I am aware of the subject matter and emotional content of my thoughts.**

2. I am aware that I make judgments where I believe I am "right" and others are "wrong."**

3. It is easy for me to concentrate.

4. I am aware of changes in my body (breathing, muscle tension, skin moisture, etc.) in response to certain thoughts.

5. I notice that my perceptions of the world are colored by my thoughts at any given time.**

6. I notice that my thoughts are influenced by my environment at any given time.

*Section 6. 4. Crying over a loss or sad event is an important discharge of emotional energy. It is, however, sometimes used as a manipulative tool, or as a substitute expression of anger. Many males in particular have been erroneously taught that it is not OK to cry.

**Section 7. 1. It is possible to be thinking many thoughts and not notice their theme or emotional direction. The ability to observe thoughts can lead to greater problem solving abilities and peace of mind.

2. We all seem to make internal judgments (play "right-wrong games") most of the time. Rather than eliminating it, being conscious of this phenomenon and not taking it too seriously allows most of us to live more pleasantly.

5. Being aware of our internal distortions of perceptions can allow us to step back and re-assess a situation more objectively when it is important to do so.

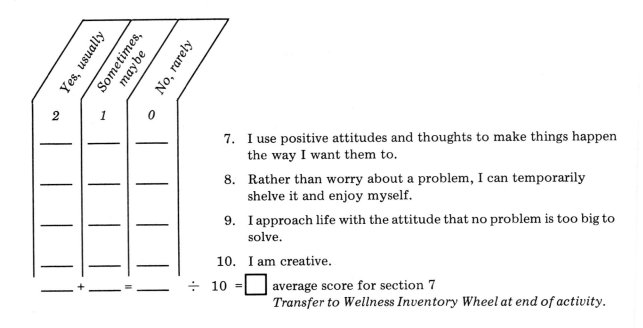

7. I use positive attitudes and thoughts to make things happen the way I want them to.

8. Rather than worry about a problem, I can temporarily shelve it and enjoy myself.

9. I approach life with the attitude that no problem is too big to solve.

10. I am creative.

_____ + _____ = _____ ÷ 10 = ☐ average score for section 7
Transfer to Wellness Inventory Wheel at end of activity.

SECTION 8—WELLNESS, PLAYING AND WORKING

1. I enjoy expressing myself through art, dance, music, drama, sports, etc., and make time to do it.

2. I enjoy spending time without planned or structured activities and make time to do it.

3. I am aware of the value of play for adults.*

4. I can approach tasks from a playful point of view.

5. At times, I allow myself to do "nothing."*

6. The work I do for income is rewarding to me.

7. I have people around me who support my playfulness.

8. I have at least one hobby or area of interest which makes no demands on me.

9. I am satisfied with my abilities to work.

10. I am satisfied with my abilities to play.

_____ + _____ = _____ ÷ 10 = ☐ average score for section 8
Transfer to Wellness Inventory Wheel at end of activity.

*Section 8. 3. Play and laughter allow the more creative self-renewing parts of our beings to emerge. Engaging in unfamiliar forms of play can reveal the self-imposed limitations we have established during childhood to protect ourselves from things we once feared.
5. Doing "nothing" often accesses the creative and non-verbal parts of you, and from another perspective, that is "everything."

SECTION 9—WELLNESS AND COMMUNICATING

Yes, usually 2	*Sometimes, maybe* 1	*No, rarely* 0	
___	___	___	1. I can introduce a difficult topic and stay with it until I've received a satisfactory response from the other person.
___	___	___	2. I enjoy silence.
___	___	___	3. I consider my thoughts and feelings with care before responding to others.
___	___	___	4. I communicate clearly with friends and family.
___	___	___	5. I assert myself to get what I need rather than feel resentment towards others for taking advantage of me.
___	___	___	6. I admit my mistakes to others when I am aware of them.
___	___	___	7. I am a good listener.
___	___	___	8. I don't interrupt or finish others' sentences for them.
___	___	___	9. I let go of mental labels and judgments I attach to persons and things in my environment, and instead see them for what they are.
___	___	___	10. I am aware of the psychological "games" I play with others.*

___ + ___ = ___ ÷ 10 = ☐   average score for section 9

Transfer to Wellness Inventory Wheel at end of activity.

SECTION 10—WELLNESS AND SEX

___	___	___	1. I feel comfortable touching and exploring my body.
___	___	___	2. I think it's OK to masturbate if one chooses to do so.
___	___	___	3. My sexual education is adequate.
___	___	___	4. I feel good about the degree of closeness I have with men in my life.
___	___	___	5. I feel good about the degree of closeness I have with women in my life.

*Section 9. 10. Psychological games as defined by Eric Berne in *Games People Play* are complex unconscious manipulations which result in the players getting negative attention and feeling bad.

Yes, usually	Sometimes maybe	No, rarely
2	1	0
____	____	____
____	____	____
____	____	____
____	____	____
____	____	____

6. I am content with my level of sexual activity.*

7. I fully experience the various stages of lovemaking rather than focus on an orgasm.*

8. I experience a desire to grow closer to other people.

9. I am aware of the difference between loving someone and needing someone's love.

10. I am able to love others without dominating or being dominated by them.

____ + ____ = ____ ÷ 10 = ☐ average score for section 10
Transfer to Wellness Inventory Wheel at end of activity.

SECTION 11—WELLNESS AND FINDING MEANING

____	____	____
____	____	____
____	____	____
____	____	____
____	____	____
____	____	____
____	____	____
____	____	____
____	____	____
____	____	____

1. I think that my life has meaning and direction, though I may not always see it clearly.

2. I think my life is challenging and exciting.

3. I have goals and objectives in my life.

4. I think I am achieving my goals.

5. I am able to talk about the death of someone close to me with family and friends.

6. I am able to talk about my death with family and friends.

7. I am prepared for and unafraid of death.**

8. I see my death as a step in my evolution.

9. I look forward to the future as an opportunity for further growth.

10. I live in the "here and now" rather than in the past or future.**

____ + ____ = ____ ÷ 10 = ☐ average score for section 11
Transfer to Wellness Inventory Wheel at end of activity.

*Section 10. 6. Including the choice to have no sexual activity.

7. A common problem for many people is overemphasis on performance and orgasm, rather than enjoying a close sensual feeling with their partner, regardless of orgasm.

**Section 11. 7. Seeing your death as a stage of growth and preparing yourself consciously is an important part of finding meaning in your life.

10. This does not imply disregarding either past or future, but seeing both in the context of your present reality. Many people live in memories of the past or fantasy worlds of the future, and are not partaking of present time reality.

SECTION 12—WELLNESS AND TRANSCENDING

Yes, usually 2	Sometimes maybe 1	No, rarely 0	
____	____	____	1. I perceive problems as opportunities for growth.
____	____	____	2. I experience synchronistic events in my life (coincidences which appear to have no cause-effect relationship but happen more often than chance would dictate).*
____	____	____	3. I believe there are dimensions of reality beyond verbal description or human comprehension.
____	____	____	4. Confusion and paradox seem a necessary part of my growth though I may at times not be comfortable with them.
____	____	____	5. The concept of "god" has a personal definition and meaning to me.
____	____	____	6. I experience a sense of wonder and awe when I contemplate the universe.
____	____	____	7. I have abundant expectancy rather than specific expectations.
____	____	____	8. I do not pressure others to accept my beliefs.
____	____	____	9. I use the messages interpreted from my dreams to better live my waking life.
____	____	____	10. I enjoy practicing a spiritual discipline or allowing time to sense the presence of a greater force in guiding my passage through life.

____ + ____ = ____ ÷ 10 = ☐ average score for section 12
Transfer to Wellness Inventory Wheel at end of activity.

THE WELLNESS INVENTORY WHEEL

Copy your average scores from each section into the square next to its heading around the index circle on the next page. Fill in the corresponding amount of each pie-section using the scales provided. The scale begins at the center with 0.0 and reaches the edge at 2.0 The dotted circle corresponds to 1.0.

*Section 12. 2. Post Einsteinian physics (quantum mechanics, Bell's Theorum, etc.) indicate that the principle of causality (something is always caused by something else) may be as limited as Newton's theories of mechanics, and that we must expand our view to see that everything in the universe is connected to everything else, regardless of the space and time intervening.

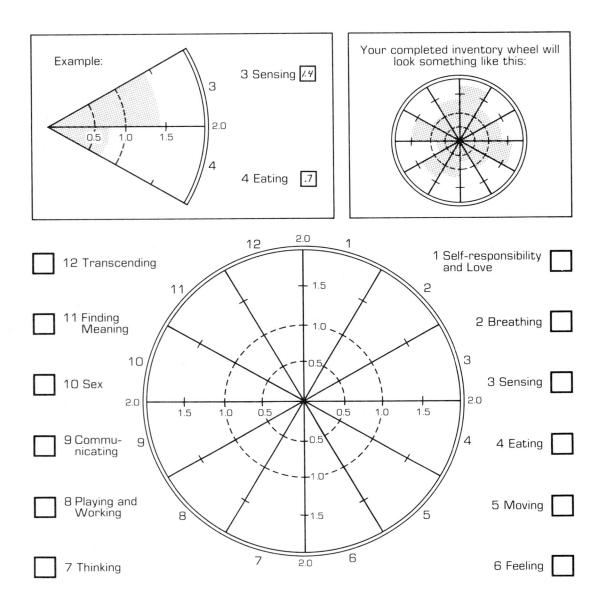

Example:

3 Sensing [1.4]

4 Eating [.7]

Your completed inventory wheel will look something like this:

12 Transcending ☐

11 Finding Meaning ☐

10 Sex ☐

9 Communicating ☐

8 Playing and Working ☐

7 Thinking ☐

1 Self-responsibility and Love ☐

2 Breathing ☐

3 Sensing ☐

4 Eating ☐

5 Moving ☐

6 Feeling ☐

Now that you have completed the Wellness Inventory, study the Wheel's shape and balance. How smoothly would it turn? What does it tell you? Are there any surprises in this for you? How does it feel to you? What don't you like about it? What do you like about it? Use it as a guide to furthering your wellness and have a great journey!

20

Identifying Personal Perceptions and Fears Regarding AIDS

Eight issues that influence health care providers who work with persons with AIDS have been frequently identified in the literature. These issues are:

1. Fear of the unknown (about the cause of the disease, its means of transmission, methods to alter its course, and even the population at risk for contracting it)

2. Fear of contagion (about contagion by proximity or of being contaminated and passing on the contamination to family and friends)

3. Fear of dying and of death (about one's own mortality, or the mortality of family and friends)

4. Denial of helplessness (difficulty in acknowledging the inability to control the course of the illness; experiencing personal failure, guilt, or burnout)

5. Homophobia (fear of homosexuality may result in refusing to work with gay clients, or in acts of hostility toward them)

6. Overidentification (investing unrealistic amounts of time and energy in the client; fusing personal needs and professional responsibilities; homosexual health providers are particularly vulnerable to overidentification)

7. Anger ("blaming the victim" because of fear, helplessness, or guilt; prevents empathy and being emotionally available to the client; or, striking out against the political and moralistic tones surrounding the AIDS epidemic and viewing the client as a means to a political end)

8. Need for professional omnipotence (when the client threatens the health care worker's expertise and power by not recognizing or appreciating the worker's role)

DISCUSSION GUIDELINES

In a group discuss the following in relation to these eight issues:

1. What are the possible ways in which these issues can be disguised and experienced as something else?

2. To which issues are you personally vulnerable?

3. Construct a peer-support system for nurses working with AIDS clients.

21

Attitudes and Beliefs about Substance Abuse

This exercise is useful in identifying your feelings, concerns, and opinions about clients with substance abuse problems. There are no "right" or "wrong" answers. Please be candid in your responses. Read each statement carefully and check (√) whether you:

1. Strongly disagree

2. Disagree

3. Neither agree nor disagree

4. Agree

5. Strongly agree

Question	Strongly agree	Agree	Neither agree nor disagree	Disagree	Strongly disagree
1. Poverty and poor environment are causes of substance abuse.	5	4	3	2	1
2. The substance abuser is a victim of circumstance.	5	4	3	2	1
3. If a substance abuser's environment is changed, use of drugs or alcohol will diminish.	5	4	3	2	1
4. Substance abuse is a symptom of an underlying emotional disturbance.	5	4	3	2	1
5. The main goal of drug abuse treatment is to gain insight about the reasons a person uses drugs.	5	4	3	2	1

Source: Questionnaire adapted from Faltz BG, Rinaldi J: *AIDS and Substance Abuse: A Training Manual for Health Care Professionals* (San Francisco: University of California, 1987), p. 26.

6. Drug or alcohol abuse results from an inability to cope with life's problems.	5	4	3	2	1
7. What substance abusers need is advice to quit or cut down on their use.	5	4	3	2	1
8. Substance abuse is a moral issue.	5	4	3	2	1
9. Jail sentences for possession of narcotics are more effective in curbing drug abuse than are drug diversion treatment programs.	5	4	3	2	1
10. A substance abuser has a chronic, progressive illness.	5	4	3	2	1
11. Alcoholism may have a biological basis.	5	4	3	2	1
12. Addiction can't be cured.	5	4	3	2	1

EXPLANATION OF SCORING

Compare your score to the description below to categorize your view of substance abuse. The current belief is that of the "disease concept."

Questions	Score	Model of Substance Abuse
1–3	Total score over 9	Problem with society/environment
4–6	Total score over 9	Result of mental disorder
7–9	Total score over 9	Moral problem
10–12	Total score over 9	Chronic, progressive disease

DISCUSSION GUIDELINES

After each of you has arrived at a score, discuss how your attitudes and beliefs regarding the four models of substance abuse are likely to influence:

1. Your assessment of persons who abuse substances

2. The nursing diagnoses you select

3. How you plan for the client's care

4. What nursing interventions you select

5. How you evaluate the effectiveness of your plan of care

22

Attitudes and Beliefs about the Substance Abuser with an HIV-Related Diagnosis

This exercise is useful in identifying your feelings, concerns, and opinions about clients with substance abuse problems and an HIV-related diagnosis. There are no "right" or "wrong" answers. Please be candid in your responses. Read each statement carefully and check (√) whether you:

1. Strongly disagree

2. Disagree

3. Neither agree nor disagree

4. Agree

5. Strongly agree

Question	Strongly agree	Agree	Neither agree nor disagree	Disagree	Strongly disagree
1. Once a person is infected with HIV there is no point in initiating drug abuse treatment	5	4	3	2	1
2. Substance abuse is not prevalent in women.	5	4	3	2	1
3. You can only help a person with a drug problem if they initiate a request for treatment.	5	4	3	2	1
4. It is difficult to be sympathetic to IV drug users who get AIDS.	5	4	3	2	1
5. Drug addicts are less concerned about their health than others.	5	4	3	2	1

Source: Questionnaire adapted from Faltz BG, Rinaldi J: *AIDS and Substance Abuse: A Training Manual for Health Care Professionals* (San Francisco: University of California, 1987), pp. 29–30.

6.   Drug abusers, as patients, usually
     request pain medications whether they
     need it or not.

5	4	3	2	1

7.   Drug abusers who are chronic
     complainers need not be taken
     seriously when they complain of
     discomfort.

5	4	3	2	1

8.   Transfusion recipients and children
     are the innocent victims of AIDS.

5	4	3	2	1

9.   If drugs were made legal, violent
     crime would decrease.

5	4	3	2	1

10. It is difficult to be sympathetic to
     homosexuals who get AIDS.

5	4	3	2	1

11. No more than 10% of hospital
     admissions results from drug or
     alcohol abuse.

5	4	3	2	1

12. Dealing with alcoholism or drug abuse
     behavior is beyond the scope of nursing
     practice.

5	4	3	2	1

13. A nurse should have the right to refuse
     care to an AIDS patient.

5	4	3	2	1

14. The difference between use and abuse
     of drugs is in the amount used.

5	4	3	2	1

15. A nurse should have the right to refuse
     care to a drug abuse patient.

5	4	3	2	1

16. Alcoholism is not as serious a problem
     as drug abuse.

5	4	3	2	1

17. Cocaine is not as dangerous as the
     media makes it seem.

5	4	3	2	1

18. A person who commits a crime "under
     the influence" of alcohol or drugs
     should not be held responsible for it.

5	4	3	2	1

19. Drug or alcohol abuse in a parent
     should be hidden from the children to
     protect them.

5	4	3	2	1

20. The relationship between physical or
     sexual abuse and the use of drugs or
     alcohol is negligible.

5	4	3	2	1

EXPLANATION OF SCORING

Add your total score and compare it to the description below.

Point score	Ease in working with substance abusers with an HIV-related diagnosis
1–20	Generally at ease in working with substance abusers. Interactions tend to be therapeutic.
21–40	Relatively at ease in working with substance abusers with HIV. May benefit from further reading list to increase knowledge.
41–80	Have some discomfort in working with substance abusers with HIV. May benefit from further reading to increase knowledge and comfort level.
81–100	May have considerable fear or discomfort in working with substance abusers with HIV. Do not give up! Your honesty and candor are gifts that can help you learn more about both AIDS and substance abuse. Increased knowledge can lead to more successful interventions with this population.

DISCUSSION GUIDELINES

After each of you has arrived at a total score, discuss how your attitudes and beliefs regarding working with a substance abuser with an HIV-related diagnosis are likely to influence:

1.   Your assessments of these clients

2.   The nursing diagnosis you select

3.   How you plan for the client's care

4.   What nursing interventions you select

5.   How you evaluate the effectiveness of your plan of care

23

Behavior and Alcoholism

This activity is designed to make you aware of your attitudes toward the use of alcohol in a variety of situations. Many factors may influence your specific reactions to these statements—for example, current alcohol use patterns, parental influence, past experiences, peer pressure. Becoming more aware of your feelings should help you to understand your behavior a little better.

DIRECTIONS

Following are seven behavioral situations involving the use of alcoholic beverages. Please circle the number on the Acceptable—Unacceptable continuum that most closely approximates your reaction.

1. A teenage, high school student is allowed to have several glasses of beer during a party for family friends given by his parents in their own home. He begins to laugh loudly and interrupts several conversations with his antics.

   ACCEPTABLE   1   2   3   4   5   6   7   8   9   10   UNACCEPTABLE

2. Many parents view a holiday like New Year's as a joyous time to celebrate. They would probably deny the youngest children at a party the privilege of consuming wine or other alcoholic beverages. However, they might allow the older children to participate. The extent to which they participate would be determined by the parents, based on their interpretation of the word "enough."

   ACCEPTABLE   1   2   3   4   5   6   7   8   9   10   UNACCEPTABLE

3. John is twenty-six years old, single, and an instructor at a state university. He comes into class "half-loaded" because his girlfriend gave him a hard time. He is a little untidy and he uses swear words instead of his normal manner. To many of the students in his class who are drinkers he is the "coolest" teacher they have ever had. They don't care if he is drunk.

Source: Adapted from *Current Health Problems: Resource and Test Questions*, by John Gay. Published 1979 by W.B. Saunders Company. Reprinted by permission Holt, Rinehart, & Winston, C.B.S. College Publishing.

There is definitely a positive reaction from those students. On the other hand, other students, including those who do not drink, are in class that day to learn the new assignment that was given the day before and are annoyed by John's behavior. How would *you* rate John's behavior?

ACCEPTABLE   1   2   3   4   5   6   7   8   9   10   UNACCEPTABLE

4.   A priest drinks wine during Mass.

ACCEPTABLE   1   2   3   4   5   6   7   8   9   10   UNACCEPTABLE

5.   The first day of finals is over and Pete, who is twenty-two years old, has just finished two tough exams. His final exam comes on the last day so he has four days of leisure before he hits the books again. Tonight Pete is celebrating with the boys in his apartment. All of Peter's friends are over twenty-one years of age. Earlier on this day Pete bought three quarts of beer for the party. When his friends arrive, the celebration begins. There is no wildness nor loud behavior, and their conduct is not out of the ordinary. After two hours of drinking the men want more beer. Pete is the only one that owns a car so Pete is elected to go out and buy some more.

ACCEPTABLE   1   2   3   4   5   6   7   8   9   10   UNACCEPTABLE

6.   Joe is a successful businessman. Sometimes the pressure gets to Joe and he goes out and gets drunk as a release. He drives home usually at excessive speeds and blames his family for things not going right with him. Within a short time Joe is in a fury and starts throwing anything he can get his hands on, often striking and injuring his wife and son. Finally, in exhaustion Joe falls into a stupor leaving his wife and son to be cared for by the neighbors.

ACCEPTABLE   1   2   3   4   5   6   7   8   9   10   UNACCEPTABLE

7.   A young couple are dating, enjoying dancing, meeting their friends, and running around until 1:30 AM each morning. Each drinks. On certain occasions and under certain conditions they will become involved in "serious" drinking. In public their conversations tend to become quite loud, yet never angry. Neither of them has ever missed work because of the late hours or hang-overs.

ACCEPTABLE   1   2   3   4   5   6   7   8   9   10   UNACCEPTABLE

DISCUSSION GUIDELINES

Divide into groups of five and discuss the following:

1.   Do you find any inconsistencies or contradictions between your opinion about the behavior described and *your* actual behavior?

2.   Compare and discuss the similarities and differences in your responses and those of classmates.

3.   How might your attitudes toward the use of alcohol affect your behavior as a professional nurse in a psychiatric or mental health setting? In a general hospital setting? In a community health agency?

24

Are You a "Rescuer"?

DIRECTIONS

Answer the following questions by writing a "Yes" or a "No" in the space at the right:

1. Do you feel your patients aren't appreciative enough of your help? _____

2. Do you pay more attention to your patients' needs than to your own needs? _____

3. Do you feel best when you are helping other people? _____

4. Do you feel responsible for other people's happiness? _____

5. Do you have difficulty letting other people come to their own decisions or voice opinions that do not agree with your own beliefs? _____

6. Do you have difficulty allowing other people to take risks or try new behaviors? _____

7. Do you always feel obligated to respond to anyone who seems to need help? _____

8. Does a large portion of your job satisfaction and personal well-being depend on your patients improving? _____

9. Are there personal needs of yours that are being met through your job that should be met outside of work? _____

EXPLANATION OF SCORING

Each question answered in the affirmative indicates rescuer belief or behavior.

Source: Adapted from Smythe EEM: *Surviving Nursing* (Addison-Wesley, 1987), pp. 141–142.

DISCUSSION GUIDELINES

In a small group discuss the old adage "You can lead a horse to water but you can't make him drink." Reformulate this adage into five different guidelines that can help nurses to better understand and avoid playing the rescuer role. Try to use as many of the following words as possible in the guidelines you formulate:

autonomy	obligation	indispensable
autocratic	responsibility	rely
power	dependency	risk
rejection	self-actualization	frustration
helpless	anxious	resentment
right	failure	

25

Stress Inoculation: Coping with Irrational, Disturbing Self-Talk

Since we all talk to ourselves, we might as well learn how to talk in ways that are helpful. The more you are aware of your distorted thinking and irrational beliefs and how these beliefs influence your self-talk, the better you will be able to control your unpleasant emotional responses to stressors. There are enough stressors in life and in nursing without your creating more personal stress from the way you talk to yourself.

DIRECTIONS:

Select a particularly stressful work situation you must deal with frequently. As you think about the situation and imagine facing it again, make statements to yourself that diffuse the situation's ability to cause you anticipatory anxiety. These are called preparation statements.

The following are examples of what you might say to yourself before an upcoming stressful event:

Don't worry, I'll be able to handle it.

I've handled worse things than this. It'll be OK.

Just think it through. Plan how to attack it and soon it'll be over.

Other people have lived through it and come out fine. So will I!

Next, imagine the steps necessary to get through the stressful events—what actually must be done. Imagine the situation as clearly and vividly as possible. This time instead of imagining you are *going* to do something, imagine that you are actually doing it. Think of things to tell yourself that will calm you as you confront the situation.

I'm in control here. Just take a few deep breaths and relax.

All I have to do is take one step at a time.

Focus on what I'm doing. If I don't pay attention to my fears, they can't stop me.

Source: Smythe EEM: *Surviving Nursing* (Addison-Wesley, 1984), pp. 187–188.

Hey, I'm doing it. It's coming along fine.

No need to be perfect. Just do the best I can.

As you imagine yourself doing the dreaded thing, you will probably notice uncomfortable feelings associated with the stress response syndrome. At this time you need calming statements. Here are a few suggestions:

Yes, I feel a little anxious. That's normal and can help me think more clearly.

I don't need to be totally relaxed; a little fear is OK. This is a new experience.

Pay attention to what I'm doing. That will stop these scary thoughts.

This will be over in a second.

If I really get overwhelmed, there is always _____ to bail me out.

Once you've survived the situation and it's over in your fantasy, reinforce your accomplishments by making self-reinforcing statements such as:

Wait till I tell _____ how I handled this!

I was great! Give me an A for the attempt.

Practice makes perfect. Sure I was a little uncomfortable, but I'm just beginning.

Only goes to show I can do anything I put my mind to.

Once you've imagined yourself through all four steps with the supportive self-statements, pick a few more upsetting, stressful situations and go through the same process until the coping self-talk comes naturally and feels familiar. Now you're ready to take on a live situation, to practice stress inoculation in vivo. As you encounter the situation, say the self-statements. If you notice tension or signs of anxiety, see these as signals alerting you to use one of your relaxation techniques. If you feel over your head at any point, give yourself permission to retrench and leave, if necessary. Above all else see the exercise as a learning experience—you don't need to be perfect. You are unlearning negative thought patterns that have developed over a long period of time. You'll need to be patient and kind to yourself as you slowly unlearn the stressful habits of irrational disturbing self-talk.

Part Two

PSYCHOSOCIAL NURSING ASSESSMENTS, STRATEGIES, AND SKILLS

26

Genius Forecasting in the Nursing Literature

Individuals such as Aldous Huxley from the past and Alvin Toffler and John Naisbett of the present stand out as genius forecasters. Leaders in nursing also have the ability to visualize nursing's future, based on their knowledge of the past.

Serious mental health professionals need to consider the implication of futuristic insights. They also need to be alert to the innate human ability to follow the rhythms and patterns of events, to sense relationships and changes, and thereby predict and shape the nature of the future.

DIRECTIONS

Find four or five major nursing journals for the months of December or January of this year. Browse through what the nursing geniuses, or recognized leaders, wrote about the future. Make a list of ten items that describe the future. Rank them according to priority by numbering from 1 to 10 in order of frequency found in the literature. Develop a synopsis for yourself of what the leaders in nursing are saying about the future. Describe what the nursing scene will be.

Priority   *Forecast*

_____   a. _____

_____   b. _____

_____   c. _____

_____   d. _____

Source: Adapted from Henderson FC, McGettigan BO: *Managing Your Career in Nursing* (Addison-Wesley, 1986), pp. 187–192.

———————   e. ————————————————————————————————————

———————   f. ————————————————————————————————————

———————   g. ————————————————————————————————————

———————   h. ————————————————————————————————————

———————   i. ————————————————————————————————————

———————   j. ————————————————————————————————————

Based on your rated list, write your view of the future psychiatric nursing scene:———————

——

——

——

——

——

——

——

DISCUSSION GUIDELINES

In a group of four or five, develop a forecast for the future of psychiatric nursing. Your group's forecast should consist of a list of ten items ranked in priority from 1 to 10.

27

The Scientific Merit of Clinical Psychiatric Nursing Research

Psychiatric nursing practice should be based on sound nursing research rather than on intuition, trial and error, or authority and tradition. As you read nursing journals, you will want to think about which clinical studies had scientific merit and possible utility for your clinical practice.

DIRECTIONS

Read the published clinical research study summarized in one of the nursing research notes in Wilson and Kneisl's *Psychiatric Nursing 3rd Edition*. Analyze the article based on Fawcett's* (1982) list of questions:

1. Has the original study been replicated?

2. If so, are the findings similar in a variety of situations?

3. Is corroboration of the findings in clinical situations done with actual clients who receive nursing care?

4. What was the risk or benefit of the nursing action tested in the study?

5. Does the study focus on a significant clinical practice problem?

6. Do nurses have clinical control over study variables?

7. Is it feasible to implement the nursing action in the real world?

8. What is the cost of implementing the nursing action?

9. What contribution to direct health status does the nursing action make?

10. What overall contribution to nursing knowledge does the study make?

*Fawcett J: Utilization of nursing research findings. *Image* June 1982; 14:57–59.

Source: Wilson H S, Hutchinson S A: *Applying Nursing Research: A Resource Book* (Addison-Wesley, 1986), p. 28.

DISCUSSION GUIDELINES

Discuss the following questions in a small group of colleagues or fellow students:

1. Does (or do) the author (or authors) of the article give enough information for you to answer all of Fawcett's questions?

2. If not, for which questions do you require more information?

3. Which of Fawcett's questions are the easiest to answer?

28

Sources of Psychiatric Nursing Research Problems

Personal experience, patterns or trends in clinical practice, somebody else's completed research reports, and your intellectual and scientific interests are all valid sources of research problems in psychiatric nursing. Recognition of these sources is one way to make you aware of potential research problems.

DIRECTIONS

The sources of research problems just mentioned are listed at the left below. Think about each source and write an example in the column at the right from your own psychiatric nursing experience.

SOURCES OF RESEARCH PROBLEMS	EXAMPLE
1. Experience a. Wishes and desires	

Source: Wilson H S, Hutchinson S A: *Applying Nursing Research: A Resource Book* (Addison-Wesley, 1987), pp. 78–80.

b. Complaints

c. Questions

2. Patterns or trends

3. Completed research (that is, reported research, case studies, clinical descriptions)

4. Your intellectual and scientific interests

DISCUSSION GUIDELINES

Discuss your examples with your colleagues or fellow students. If you had all the time in the world and access to unlimited resources, which of your examples would you choose to study? Why?

29

Client Assessment Form

DIRECTIONS

Using data from your process recordings, complete the following guide for assessing your client's assets and coping deficits.

FOCUS	ASSETS	PROBLEMS

A. Ability to assume responsibilities for self-care
 	
  1. Physical care
 	
    a. Personal hygiene
 	
    b. Maintenance of body functions
 	
  2. Observance of common safety measures
 	
  3. Use of manual skills		

Source: Janet A. Simmons, *The Nurse-Client Relationship in Mental Health Nursing* (Philadelphia: W. B. Saunders Co., 1976), pp. 154-57.

FOCUS	ASSETS	PROBLEMS
4. Use of cognitive skills		
5. Use of skill in interpersonal relations		
a. With relatives		
b. With peers		
c. With authority figures		
d. With nurse		
B. Accomplishment of developmental level tasks		
1. Trust		
2. Autonomy		
3. Initiative		
4. Industry		

FOCUS	*ASSETS*	*PROBLEMS*
5. Identity		
6. Intimacy		
7. Generativity		
8. Integrity		
C. Communication		
1. Accuracy		
2. Clarity		
3. Descriptive ability		
4. Preciseness		
5. Use of concrete terms		
6. Use of abstract terms		

FOCUS	ASSETS	PROBLEMS
7. Use of logical associations		
D. Perception of reality 1. View of self 2. Body image 3. Interpretation of environment 4. Interpretation of others in environment		

30

Milieu Assessment Tool

DIRECTIONS

Using data assembled in your process recording notes, complete the following guide to assess the strengths and weaknesses of your client's milieu.

MILIEU ASPECT	*STRENGTHS*	*WEAKNESSES*
Provisions for support of physical needs		
Provisions for support of physical comfort		
Provisions for support of psychological comfort		

Source: Janet A. Simmons, *The Nurse-Client Relationship in Mental Health Nursing* (Philadelphia: W. B. Saunders Co., 1976), pp. 162-63.

MILIEU ASPECT	STRENGTHS	WEAKNESSES
Provisions for support of sociocultural needs (affiliation etc.)		
Personal space		
Personal time		
Possibility of change		
Greatest asset		
Greatest weakness		

31

Diagramming Interactions in Milieus

The simplest technique for studying the social structure of a hospital unit milieu is to use diagrams such as figure 1 (next page). A major purpose of assessing a milieu this way is to help the client take advantage of the therapeutic possibilities on a psychiatric unit. In order to promote healthy socialization, staff members first need to study the unit's existing social structure.

People often become psychiatric clients because they have not learned to live comfortably in social relationships with others. They need experience in effective social living, and, in many hospitals, the psychiatric unit has become the therapeutic community that furnishes this experience. Nurses, aides, and attendants, who, in effect, live with the clients, must use the everyday experiences of the clients' lives on the unit—eating, getting up and going to sleep, meeting personal hygiene needs, working, talking, and playing together—as therapy. This is therapy with twenty-four-hour-a-day possibilities. The unit must become a setting in which there is consideration for each person's needs, where there is acceptance, understanding, and the opportunity for emotional growth.

As a nurse, you need to be constantly aware of the social relationships on the unit and the part you can play in helping the clients to improve them.

DIRECTIONS

To study the social structure of your unit, make a series of diagrams of interactions you observe at different times and places on the unit, and answer questions such as the following:

1. Who is the leader? Are there two leaders? Is there a hostile leader?

2. Who belongs to each existing group?

3. Who are the fringe members?

4. Who are the isolates?

Source: Reprinted by Permission. American Journal of Nursing, 10 Columbus Circle, New York, NY 10019.

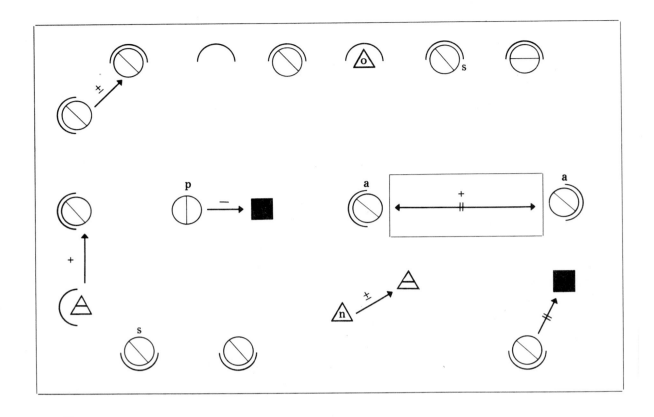

Key:

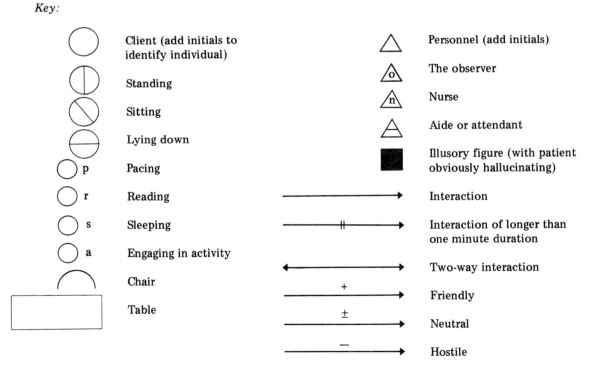

Figure 1. Sample interaction diagram of an inpatient milieu

5.   Where does the most socializing occur: in the dining room, dayrooms, occupational therapy, outdoors, etc.?

6.   Is there competition among the clients to be the "sickest"?

7.   What persons or what activities promote friendly interaction?

8.   What persons or activities block friendly interaction?

9.   With which patients do personnel spend most time and effort?

10.   What clients need individual help before they can interact independently with others and become a part of the unit society?

11.   What opportunities are there to foster competence in group living—client government, remotivation groups, discussion groups, activity groups? Can you handle discussions on such topics as family relationships, managing angry feelings, making friends, working and competing with others, attitudes, and authority figures? Can you help each client to think "we" instead of "I"?

USING INTERACTION DIAGRAMS

Diagraming can be of inestimable value in helping you to answer these questions. It is of particular value when a new client is introduced, and the therapeutic team wishes to study the newcomer's manner of relating to or withdrawing from the group and the role he or she plays in the unit. Diagraming can help you to capitalize on client "clusters"—it may reveal clients who exclude themselves or are excluded. However, a single diagram made at one particular time has little significance. Only when you have made many diagrams at different times of day, on different days, and in different places over a period of time, can you draw valid conclusions about recurring patterns.

The interaction diagram can be used by all levels of nursing personnel. As you continue to use it and discuss the findings it reveals with other personnel, you will all become acutely aware of those clients who need the most help in interacting with others. Clients who have the greatest problems in interacting, because they either withdraw or relate in a hostile fashion, can be selected for more intensive individual nurse-client relationships. Personnel who avoid relating to clients or who relate nontherapeutically can be counseled. Client leadership potential can be discovered and encouraged. You can evaluate objectively which activities promote friendly interaction and which ones hinder it. Clients can learn the technique of diagraming and can chart their group progress from social disorganization to social integration. The unit milieu is not static but dynamic and changing. Only if you keep aware of this factor can you introduce constructive changes.

32
Literature as a Means to Understanding Total Institutions

This activity stimulates you to explore the characteristics of total institutions and the processes of institutionalization by critically analyzing fiction and nonfiction works on these subjects.

DIRECTIONS

Read the following:

1. Erving Goffman, *Asylums* (Garden City, N.Y.: Doubleday Anchor Books, 1961), pp. xiii, 1-124.

2. Ken Kesey, *One Flew Over the Cuckoo's Nest* (New York: New American Library, Signet Edition, 1966).

DISCUSSION GUIDELINES

Engage in a small group discussion of the following questions:

1. In the total institution as discussed by Goffman, enforced activities are brought together into a single rational plan purportedly designed to fulfill the official aim of the institution. What do you think the ultimate aim of Kesey's "Big Nurse" is, based on what you observe about the enforced activities on her ward?

2. In total institutions, Goffman asserts, there is a basic split between a large managed group called *inmates* and a small supervisory staff. What in Kesey's novel might symbolize this split or distance?

3. A characteristic of total institutions is a demoralized work system. Can you cite an example of such a system from Kesey's novel?

4. In our society, total institutions, according to Goffman's framework, are the forcing houses for changing persons: each institution is an experiment about what can be done with the self. This idea is discussed to a great extent by Bromden in *Cuckoo's Nest.*

What is Bromden's name for the concept? Can you cite some evidence to support it from Kesey's novel?

5. Upon entering a total institution, inmates are immediately stripped of their "presenting culture." This is the first in a series of abasements, degradations, and humiliations of the self they undergo. What about McMurphy's admission process captures this attempt on the part of the total institution?

6. Both Goffman and Kesey discuss admission procedures. "The new arrival allows himself to be coded into an object that can be fed into the administrative machinery of the establishment," says Goffman. What are some examples of admission procedures from *Cuckoo's Nest?*

7. Mortification, according to Goffman, occurs when inmates expose their interpersonal relationships and when they take no action when an assault is made upon a fellow inmate. An example quoted in *Asylums* is Herman Melville's description of flogging in the British navy (p. 34). Goffman comments that "all conveys a terrible hint of the omnipotent authority under which [the inmate] lives." Give a clear example of mortification in this form from *Cuckoo's Nest.*

8. Regimentation and tyranny are characteristic of total institutions. Autonomy of action is violated, and inmates are not permitted to schedule their own activities. Cite examples of this from Big Nurse's ward.

9. Goffman notes that inmates may be considered so insignificant in status by staff that they are not given even minor greetings. How does Bromden's "deafness" relate to this observation?

10. The "privilege system" of the total institution represents the framework for the inmate's personal reorganization after stripping occurs. Punishments in this system are the consequences of breaking the rules. How might McMurphy's brief withdrawal from "the battle" be considered in this context?

11. Can you think of examples in Kesey's novel of "messing up" as defined by Goffman? What were the consequences for those involved?

12. Institutional ceremonies that occur through such media as the house organ, group meetings, open house programs, and charitable performances presumably fulfill latent social functions, according to Goffman. However, he goes on to state that often there is a hint of rebellion in the role the inmates take. They use these ceremonies as opportunities in which subordinates can in some way profane superordinates. When and how does this occur in Kesey's novel?

13. Goffman comments that the contradiction between what the institution does and what its officials say it does forms the basic context of the staff's daily activity. Do you see this contradiction in *Cuckoo's Nest* when the public relations man visits the ward? How is it illustrated by what goes on in the "therapeutic group meetings"?

14. The obligation of the staff to maintain certain humane standards of treatment for inmates presents problems in itself, but a further set of characteristic problems is found in the constant conflict between humane standards and organizational efficiency. Just as personal possessions may interfere with smooth running of an institutional operation and be removed for this reason, so parts of the body may also conflict with efficient management, and the conflict may be resolved in favor of efficiency. This occurs in

Kesey's novel on a symbolic level with Billy Bibbit and more explicitly in the case of McMurphy. What happens?

15. Often the privileges and punishments that the staff mete out are phrased in language that reflects the legitimated objectives of the institution. This practice is basic to the means of social control. In these terms, how does McMurphy threaten the control of Big Nurse?

33

Observation of Nonverbal Behavior

DIRECTIONS

From your observations of a client, select an example of nonverbal behavior. Describe it on the form provided below.

Client's nonverbal behavior	
Possible meaning(s) of behavior	
Assessment of apparent reasons for behavior	

Nursing intervention	
Outcome of intervention	
Evaluation of effectiveness of intervention	
Suggested alternative intervention	

34

Life Crises Scale

Researchers Holmes and Masuda have concluded that clusters of certain life events help to make a person vulnerable to illness. They found that the events of ordinary life—such as marriage, vacation, a new job—can help to trigger illness because they require energy to cope with them and therefore reduce a person's resistance to illness.

DIRECTIONS

Using yourself or a client as the subject, place a check mark on the line to the left of each event that has occurred in the subject's life during the past year. If the event has occurred more than once, place a check mark for each occurrence.

_____ 1. Death of spouse

_____ 2. Divorce

_____ 3. Marital separation

_____ 4. Jail term

_____ 5. Death of close family member

_____ 6. Personal injury or illness

_____ 7. Marriage

_____ 8. Firing from work

_____ 9. Marital reconciliation

_____ 10. Retirement

_____ 11. Change in health of family member

_____ 12. Pregnancy

_____ 13. Sexual difficulties

_____ 14. Gain of new family member

_____ 15. Business readjustment

_____ 16. Change in financial state

_____ 17. Death of close friend

_____ 18. Change to different line of work

_____ 19. Change in number of arguments with spouse

_____ 20. Mortgage over $10,000

_____ 21. Foreclosure of mortgage or loan

_____ 22. Change in responsibilities at work

_____ 23. Son or daughter leaving home

Source: Adapted from Thomas H. Holmes and Minoru Masuda, "Psychosomatic Syndrome," _Psychology Today_, April 1972, p. 71. REPRINTED FROM PSYCHOLOGY TODAY MAGAZINE. Copyright ©1972 Ziff-Davis Publishing Company.

_____ 24. Trouble with in-laws

_____ 25. Outstanding personal achievement

_____ 26. Spouse beginning or stopping work

_____ 27. Beginning or ending school

_____ 28. Change in living conditions

_____ 29. Revision of personal habits

_____ 30. Trouble with boss

_____ 31. Change in work hours or conditions

_____ 32. Change in residence

_____ 33. Change in schools

_____ 34. Change in recreation

_____ 35. Change in church activities

_____ 36. Change in social activities

_____ 37. Mortgage or loan less than $10,000

_____ 38. Change in sleeping habits

_____ 39. Change in number of family get-togethers

_____ 40. Change in eating habits

_____ 41. Vacation

_____ 42. Christmas

_____ 43. Minor violations of the law

EXPLANATION OF SCORING

In the blanks to the right below, enter the listed mean value for each life event you have checked, and add up the values to get the subject's total score.

Event	Mean Value	
1	100	____
2	73	____
3	65	____
4	63	____
5	63	____
6	53	____
7	50	____
8	47	____
9	45	____
10	45	____
11	44	____
12	40	____
13	39	____
14	39	____
15	39	____
16	38	____
17	37	____
18	36	____

Event	Mean Value	
19	35	_____
20	31	_____
21	30	_____
22	29	_____
23	29	_____
24	29	_____
25	28	_____
26	26	_____
27	26	_____
28	25	_____
29	24	_____
30	23	_____
31	20	_____
32	20	_____
33	20	_____
34	19	_____
35	19	_____
36	18	_____
37	17	_____
38	16	_____
39	15	_____
40	15	_____
41	13	_____
42	12	_____
43	11	_____

Subject's total _____

Find the subject's life crises level among the following categories:

150-199   Mild risk

200-299   Moderate risk

300 or more Major risk

The higher the risk level, the more likely it is that the subject will encounter illness within the year. Of the subjects Holmes and Masuda studied, 37 percent in the mild risk category, 51 percent in the moderate risk category, and 79 percent in the major risk category had associated health changes.

DISCUSSION GUIDELINES

In seminar or small groups, discuss these questions:

1. What are the implications of this exercise for primary prevention? Secondary prevention? Tertiary prevention?

2. What nursing actions are possible in relation to persons in the mild risk category? The moderate risk category? The major risk category?

3. Recent research indicates that the event itself (change in health of family member), and not the valence of the event (change for the better, or change for the worse), constitutes a stressful life event because it requires adaptive or coping behavior. What are the implications of this finding?

35

Myths about Suicide

DIRECTIONS

Mark **T** for true or **F** for false on the line to the left of each of the following statements.

—— 1. Women attempt suicide more often than men.

—— 2. Only cowards and weaklings consider suicide as an alternative.

—— 3. Once suicidal, always suicidal.

—— 4. Unfortunately, suicide happens without warning.

—— 5. It is better to discuss hopeful and pleasant things with a suicidal person than it is to discuss the person's suicidal intent.

—— 6. Suicide attempts are manipulative ploys.

—— 7. The surest way to commit suicide is to turn on the gas.

—— 8. Tendencies toward suicide are inherited.

—— 9. More rich people than poor people attempt suicide.

—— 10. Only psychotic persons try to kill themselves.

—— 11. If a person talks about intending to commit suicide, he or she won't do it.

—— 12. Suicidal persons are usually intent on dying.

—— 13. Suicide is seldom attempted by intelligent persons.

—— 14. Suicide is seldom attempted by well-educated persons.

—— 15. The immediate suicide risk is over when improvement follows a suicidal crisis.

EXPLANATION OF SCORING

All of the statements are *false*. These fifteen items constitute the most frequently held myths or "old wives' tales" about suicide and suicidal persons.

DISCUSSION GUIDELINES

On a chalkboard, tabulate the responses of all the students to each question. Discuss each myth in turn, considering factors such as:

1. What in your life experience might have led you to respond as you did?

2. How might your beliefs about suicide influence your interactions and effectiveness with suicidal persons?

36

Exploring the Issues in Community Mental Health Nursing

This activity can be used as an independent assignment followed by in-class discussion or as a small group experience.

The Situation

You are one of fifteen applicants for three community mental health nurse positions recently funded by a private philanthropic foundation. The positions are in a highly respected community mental health agency located in the downtown area of a large city. Working there would provide you with exactly the kind of professional experience you desire most.

The Program Director has asked each candidate to meet with the full staff of the agency so that they can learn the position of prospective community mental health nurses on several critical issues facing the agency

For each of the issues listed:

1. Indicate your position.

2. List two reasons for taking the position you did and two reasons for rejecting an alternative position.

The Issues

1. The agency is considering two potential ways in which these funds can be used for personnel. Which course of action do you advocate assuming that combined salaries in both situations are equal?

    a. Using the funds to hire *three* community mental health nurses as originally planned, or

    b. Using the funds to hire *one* community mental health nurse and *five* indigenous non-professional mental health workers?

2. Should clients be invited to participate in case conferences?

3. Where does the responsibility of nurses lie—in providing nursing care to clients according to the A. N. A. Standards of Psychiatric and Mental Health Nursing Practice, or according to the policies and procedures of the employing agency?

4. Will using the DSM-III facilitate or obstruct the delivery of humanistic psychiatric nursing services to clients?

5. Almost all of the clients on the case load of this agency are assigned to one-to-one counselors. Many of the newer professionals on staff strongly believe that since all people have lived in families or groups that family and group therapy should be the preferred mode of treatment for all clients. Where do you stand?

6. If clients have rights, do they also have responsibilities? If a list of client rights is posted, should a list of client responsibilities be posted as well? What should be included in a list of client rights? In a list of client responsibilities?

7. Is deinstitutionalization a failure? What should be the agency position regarding deinstitutionalization and psychiatric chronicity?

8. Since financial resources to the agency have been cut back in most instances (except for the new nursing positions) where should the agency place its emphasis? On primary prevention? On secondary prevention? On tertiary prevention?

DISCUSSION GUIDELINES

Discuss your positions and rationales with:

1. The person seated next to you.

2. Your other classmates during an in-class discussion.

3. Other members of your small group in a simulated meeting with the agency staff (who may question your position or ask for further explanations).

37

Group Member Selection Interview Guide

DIRECTIONS

Complete this profile for each individual you interview who is a candidate for your therapy group. Before filling out the form the first time, duplicate sufficient copies of it for each use.

Potential Group Member Profile

Name: _____ Date of interview: _____

Age: _____ Length of interview: _____

Sex: _____

The problem as the client views it:

Behavioral descriptive data:

Expected effect of this client on other members:

Risk of client's premature termination:

Check yes or no for each item.	*YES*	*NO*
1. Denial is high		
2. Somatization is high		
3. Motivation is low		
4. Psychological-mindedness is low		
5. Physical reasons interfere (transportation, distance, scheduling conflict, etc.)		
6. Current life stress is high		
7. Client has problems with intimacy or disclosure		

Risk of premature termination from the group is determined by the number of items checked in the yes column. The more items checked yes, the greater the risk.

Recommendations for group therapy (including rationale):

_____

Group Leader(s)

DISCUSSION GUIDELINES

With your cotherapist or instructor, discuss the following questions:

1. What are your selection criteria for including a client within the group?

2. What are your impressions of each individual's motivation toward group treatment?

3. Considering your recommendations about membership for all candidates, what is the composition and balance of the group? What characteristics does the group have?

4. Based on your answers to question 3, what are your expectations about the possible initial behavior of the group as a whole and of its individual members?

38

Analysis of Group Inclusion, Control, and Affection Needs

This tool is based on the work of Schutz.* It may be used to analyze a group you are leading or another therapist's group. It can also be used for nontherapy groups.

DIRECTIONS

In the form below, give verbatim data from a group therapy session that demonstrates group members' inclusion, control, and affection needs and the therapist's responses. Analyze the data in the last column. Then answer the questions that follow the form. Complete this tool a total of three times:

1. For one of the first three sessions.
2. For one of the middle sessions.
3. For one of the final three sessions.

Before filling out the form the first time, duplicate sufficient copies of it for each use.

*See W. C. Schutz, *The Interpersonal Underworld: FIRO* (Palo Alto, Calif.: Science and Behavior Books, 1958).

VERBATIM EXAMPLE	INTERVENTION AND RATIONALE	ANALYSIS

QUESTIONS

1. Comment on the inclusion, control, or affection needs of the group members whose verbal and nonverbal behaviors are not included in the verbatim example column.

2. Comment on the inclusion, control, or affection needs of the therapist and their manifestation during this session.

3. What do these data tell you about the stage of the group?

4. Based on the preceding data and the therapist's method of dealing with inclusion, control, and affection needs, what is your prediction about the future manifestation of these needs within the group?

39

Mental Health Services in Your Community

DIRECTIONS

Using the charts below, identify the mental health services, facilities, and programs available in your community, and evaluate them, using the following code:

A = Adequate

L = Limited

I = Inadequate

Community facilities for mental health treatment:

SERVICE	AGENCY	ADMISSION WAITING TIME (WEEKS)	ASSESSMENT (A) (L) (I)
Emergency services			
Short-term care			
Day care			
Night care			
Halfway houses			

SERVICE	AGENCY	ADMISSION WAITING TIME (WEEKS)	ASSESSMENT (A) (L) (I)
Domiciliary care			
Suicide prevention			
Crisis or walk-in clinics			
Outpatient clinics			
Home follow-ups			
Sheltered workshops			
Foster care			
Patient clubs			
Prehospital screening			
Industrial mental health services			
Consultation services			
Preventive services			
Other			

Other groups and agencies having mental health programs:

GROUP	SPECIFIC PROGRAMS	ASSESSMENT (A) (L) (I)
Clergy		
Courts		
Police		
Schools		
Welfare		
Other		

Substance Abuse Addiction Services in Your Community

DIRECTIONS

Using the charts below, identify the alcoholism and drug addiction services and programs available in your community, and evaluate them, using the following code:

A = Adequate

L = Limited

I = Inadequate

Agencies providing alcoholism services and programs:

SERVICE	*AGENCY*	*ASSESSMENT (A) (L) (I)*
Education		
Counseling		
Case finding		
Inpatient treatment		
Aftercare		

SERVICE	AGENCY	ASSESSMENT (A) (L) (I)
Rehabilitation		
Employment		
Home follow-up		
Outpatient clinics		
Alcoholics Anonymous groups		
Family counseling		
Halfway houses		
Other		

Agencies providing drug addiction services and programs:

SERVICE	AGENCY	ASSESSMENT (A) (L) (I)
Education		
Counseling		
Case finding		
Inpatient treatment		

SERVICE	AGENCY	ASSESSMENT (A) (L) (I)
Aftercare		
Rehabilitation		
Employment		
Home follow-up		
Outpatient clinics		
Residential programs		
Family counseling		
Halfway houses		
Other		

41

Misuse and Abuse of Prescription Drugs

This exercise will help to determine whether your client uses prescription drugs properly.

DIRECTIONS

Ask your client to consider his or her use of prescription drugs and respond to each of the following questions. Circle the YES if the answer is true for your client and the NO if the answer is not true for your client.

Does Your Client . . .

1.	Know its name or why it was prescribed?	YES	NO
2.	Know how or when to take it to make it most effective?	YES	NO
3.	Always remember to take it?	YES	NO
4.	Take only the prescribed dosage even if he or she forgets to take it one time?	YES	NO
5.	Take doses only at proper time?	YES	NO
6.	Recognize side effects?	YES	NO
7.	Notify the physician if he or she discontinues it?	YES	NO
8.	Take the drug for the prescribed time period and avoid stretching it to make it last longer?	YES	NO
9.	Not seek a refill long after the rational need for it has disappeared?	YES	NO
10.	Dispose of old medicine to avoid self-treatment at a later time?	YES	NO
11.	Not borrow or lend medicines?	YES	NO

Source: Reprinted by permission from Stafford Cox, et al., *Wellness R.S.V.P.*, Menlo Park, CA: The Benjamin/Cummings Publishing Company, 1981, p. 28.

12. Tell the physician if he or she is taking medicine not prescribed by him or her?   YES   NO

13. Avoid taking too much, thinking that if one dose is helpful, two would be even better?   YES   NO

14. Avoid taking too much by taking duplicate medicines prescribed by two different physicians?   YES   NO

15. Avoid mixing alcohol with such drugs as tranquilizers, barbiturates, and antihistamines?   YES   NO

                                                          Total   _____

EXPLANATION OF SCORING

Your client's response to each of the questions should be yes. If your client is between the ages of eighteen and twenty-five, the chances are about one in four that he or she has misused a prescription drug. Careful use of medications helps them work more effectively and helps prevent serious side effects.

42

How Well Do You Know the Elderly?

One reason for indifference and hostility toward the aged in our society is that most people simply do not know what it is like to be old. To be sure, growing old brings changes, both within and without, and a decline in physical powers, but many of the changes people dread are myths, not facts. This short test will give you a chance to see how much you know about aging and possibly correct some misconceptions you may have had concerning the elderly.

DIRECTIONS

Circle what you think the correct answer is for each statement.

1. The majority of old persons (past age sixty-five) are senile (i.e., defective memory, disoriented, or demented).   T   F

2. All five senses tend to decline in old age.   T   F

3. Most old persons have no interest in, or capacity for sexual relations.   T   F

4. Lung capacity tends to decline in old age.   T   F

5. At least one-tenth of the aged are living in long-stay institutions like nursing homes or homes for the aged.   T   F

6. Aged drivers have fewer accidents per person than drivers under age sixty-five.   T   F

7. Most older workers cannot work as effectively.   T   F

8. About eighty percent of the aged are healthy enough to carry out their normal activities.   T   F

9. Most old persons are set in their ways and unable to change.   T   F

Source: "Facts on Aging: A Short Quiz," Erdman Palmore, Ph.D. Reprinted by permission of *The Gerontologist* Vol. 17, No. 4, 1977, pp. 315-316.

10.	The reaction time of most old persons tends to be slower.	T	F
11.	The majority of old persons are socially isolated and lonely.	T	F
12.	Older workers have fewer accidents than younger workers.	T	F
13.	The majority of older persons have incomes below the poverty level (as defined by the federal government).	T	F
14.	The majority of old persons are working or would like to have some kind of work to do.	T	F
15.	Older persons tend to become more religious as they age.	T	F

EXPLANATION OF SCORING

All the odd numbered items are false and all the even numbered are true. There is no "pass" or "fail" grade on the above test, but consider that a sample of college undergraduates scored sixty-five percent correct, graduate students eighty percent, and faculty ninety percent.

43

Guidelines for Assessing Dementia in Elderly Clients ("DEMENTIA")

DIRECTIONS

Changes in mentation among elderly clients can occur in response to physical conditions, stress, and medications. Psychiatric nurses can use the demential assessment tool below when collecting data with clients who exhibit the behavioral changes associated with dementia. Select an elderly client whose psychiatric diagnosis is dementia and use the following guidelines to collect data crucial to establishing a nursing care plan:

D	Drugs	Names of psychoactive drugs? Dosage? Interactions?
E	Emotions	Depression? Anxiety? Bereavement?
M	Metabolic/endocrine	Diabetes? Thyroid disease? Dehydration?
E	Environment	Change in living situation? Vision problems? Hearing loss? Other sensory loss?

Source: Adapted with permission from unpublished clinical teaching material used by Carol Detrich, NP, University of California: San Francisco, School of Nursing.

N	Nutrition	Anemia? Folic Acid? B_{12} deficiency? Alcoholism? Constipation? Poor dentures? Poverty? Transportation?
T	Tumor/trauma	CAT scan findings? Other test results?
I	Infection	Pulmonary? Urinary tract?
A	Acute condition	Myocardial infarction with CHF? Pulmonary emboli?

DISCUSSION

Discuss your findings in relation to the following related pieces of "clinical wisdom":

1. Elders are 23 times more likely to take psychoactive drugs than other age groups and they are susceptible to heightened sensitivity, delayed action, and confusion.

2. Among the elderly, clinicians must watch both for the dementia of depression and the depression of dementia.

3. Blood sugar level norms are based on 20 years olds. Thyroid disease in elders usually presents as hypothyroidism whether the condition is hypo or hyper. Diminished thirst is characteristic of many older adults.

4. Paranoia among elders is often associated with sensory loss.

5. Toxic delirium can result from constipation among the elderly.

6. Pituitary tumors in clients over the age of 50 often present as a vision change.

7. Elderly clients may not have a temperature elevation or increased pulse in the presence of an infection. Respiratory rate change is the best indicator of infection.

8. Change in mentation may be the first indicator of an acute illness like myocardial infarction; some of the medications used for acute conditions waste vitamin B_{12}, contribute to peripheral neuropathy, and predispose the elders to falling down.

44

Planning Nursing Interventions with Confused Elderly

DIRECTIONS

Impaired cognitive function resulting in confusion is a frequently encountered client problem among the elderly. Formulate specific nursing interventions for each of the following eight general principles for planning nursing care for such clients.

1. Establish orientation to the environment

2. Provide for safety, stability, and support in the environment

3. Reinforce the client's sense of personal identity and self-esteem

4. Modify the environment to avoid sensory monotony, sensory deprivation, and sensory overload

5. Use medications cautiously

6. Collect data concerning possible causes for increased confusion and agitation at night

7. Restore and maintain physiological functioning and prevent further decompensation

8. Demonstrate awareness that care of confused elderly people requires time, patience, and teamwork

DISCUSSION

Divide into groups of three to five and share with each other the specific nursing interventions generated under each of the general principles in this list. Consider the following questions:

1. How similar were your interventions?

2. How diverse were they?

3. Which principle was most difficult to implement in practical ways?

Source: Adapted with permission from unpublished clinical teaching material used by Carol Detrich, NP, University of California: San Francisco, School of Nursing.

45

Using Confrontation Effectively

A *confrontation* is a deliberate attempt to help another person to examine the consequences of some aspect of his or her behavior by sharing your perceptions of that behavior, its impact on you, and the inferences you draw about its motives and meaning. In an *informational* confrontation, you describe the visible behavior of another person. In an *interpretive* confrontation, you express what you think or feel about the meaning of another's behavior.

Six skills are involved in constructive confrontations:

1. The use of personal statements, *I, me, my,*

2. The use of relationship statements in which you express what you think or feel about the person with whom you are interacting,

3. The use of statements describing the visible behavior of the other person,

4. The use of descriptions of personal feelings specifying the feeling by name,

5. The use of understanding responses, such as paraphrasing and perception checking,

6. The use of constructive feedback skills.

The following learning activities offer you opportunities to practice confronting another person constructively. In each confrontation you should consciously apply the six confrontation skills. This activity is composed of three exercises that may be used separately or sequentially. Engaging in all three within a short period of time, however, may be an uncomfortably intense experience.

ROLE-PLAYING CONFRONTATIONS

Directions

1. Divide into triads. Designate one person as the confronter, another as the person being confronted, and the third as the observer.

Source: Reprinted from: John E. Jones and J. William Pfeiffer, "Confrontation: Types, Conditions, and Outcomes," THE 1973 ANNUAL HANDBOOK FOR GROUP FACILITATORS. San Diego, CA: 1973. Used with permission.

2. The group leader will assign a role-playing situation to each triad. The person being confronted plays the person described in the situation. The confronter tries to confront the other with as much authenticity and involvement as possible. The observer evaluates the effectiveness of the use of constructive confrontation, applying the six confrontation skills, as criteria.

3. After the confrontation has ended, the other two members of the triad give the confronter feedback on her or his use of the skills involved in constructive confrontation.

4. All three members switch roles and repeat the process with a different situation.

5. Again switch roles and repeat with a third situation.

Roles

The person being confronted plays the following role:

1. A person who is so "nice" that she or he is "unreal."

2. A person who constantly expresses a great deal of affection for everyone.

3. A person who jokes about other people's problems.

4. A person who frequently embarrasses others by making gross remarks and displaying bad table manners.

5. A person who is extremely shy in groups.

6. A person who often criticizes the behavior of others.

Discussion Guidelines

In the group as a whole, consider the following questions:

1. What did you learn about how you may confront other individuals more effectively?

2. What were your reactions to the exercise?

RELATIONSHIP CONFRONTATIONS

This exercise gives you an opportunity to use confrontation to improve the quality of your relationships.

Directions

1. Select a person with whom you have a good relationship. Between you, discuss the following issues, using the skills involved in constructive confrontation:

    a. "The things you do that most block our relationship are . . ."

    b. "The things you could do to improve our relationship are . . ."

2. At the end of fifteen minutes stop. Then choose another person with whom you have a good relationship. Again discuss these two issues.

3. At the end of fifteen minutes stop. Repeat the exercise with a third partner with whom you have a good relationship.

Discussion Guidelines

In the group as a whole, discuss your reactions to the exercise.

GOING AROUND THE CIRCLE

This exercise provides an opportunity for you to practice good confrontation skills with everyone in the group.

Directions

1. If you wish to participate in the exercise, form a circle with the other participants.

2. One at a time, you walk around the circle, stopping in front of each person. Look directly at the person, touch the person, and tell the person how you feel about her or him and your relationship.

Discussion Guidelines

After every participant has gone around the circle, discuss the following questions as a group:

1. What were your reactions to the exercise?

2. What did you learn about yourself and the other participants from it?

3. What could you do to improve your relationships with the other members of the group?

After completing all three exercises, you may wish to do a self-assessment in terms of confrontation skills. Check the appropriate statement:

——— I have mastered constructively confronting other individuals.

——— I need more work on constructively confronting other individuals.

46

Understanding Silence

This tool may be used to help you understand silence in therapeutic encounters.

DIRECTIONS

In the form below, note your observations about the quality and quantity of the silence that occurs in sessions with a client and the verbal and nonverbal behavior of both client and nurse. Analyze the silences according to the guidelines that follow the form.

Complete this tool a total of five times, after reviewing your data from:

1. The first session with the client (whether individual, group, or family).

2. The second session.

3. The final session.

4. Any other two sessions.

Before filling out the form the first time, duplicate sufficient copies of it for each use.

LENGTH AND FEELING TONE OF SILENCE	VERBAL AND NONVERBAL DATA PRECEDING, DURING, AND AFTER SILENCE	NURSE RESPONSES (THOUGHTS, FEELINGS, ACTIONS)

ANALYSIS GUIDELINES

In the space below, analyze the silences by comparing therapeutic sessions. Is there a trend in terms of the client's responses? What is it? What is the significance of silence with this client? Is there a pattern to your responses? What is it? What is the significance of your pattern of responses to the client?

47

Body Ritual among the Nacirema: Cultural Awareness and Analysis

This activity stimulates you to explore the importance of magical beliefs and ritual practices in the culture of a tribe described by anthropologist Horace Miner.

DIRECTIONS

Read the following article.

Body Ritual Among the Nacirema*

Horace Miner
University of Michigan

The anthropologist has become so familiar with the diversity of ways in which different peoples behave in similar situations that he is not apt to be surprised by even the most exotic customs. In fact, if all of the logically possible combinations of behavior have not been found somewhere in the world, he is apt to suspect that they must be present in some yet undescribed tribe. This point has, in fact, been expressed with respect to clan organization by Murdock (1949:71). In this light, the magical beliefs and practices of the Nacirema present such unusual aspects that it seems desirable to describe them as an example of the extremes to which human behavior can go.

Professor Linton first brought the ritual of the Nacirema to the attention of anthropologists twenty years ago (1936:326), but the culture of this people is still very poorly understood. They are a North American group living in the territory between the Canadian Cree, the Yaqui and Tarahumare of Mexico, and the Carib and Arawak of the Antilles. Little is known of their origin, although tradition states that they came from the east. According to Nacirema mythology, their nation was originated by a culture hero, Notgnihsaw, who is otherwise known for two great feats of strength—the throwing of a piece of wampum across the river Pa-To-Mac and the chopping down of a cherry tree in which the Spirit of Truth resided.

Source: Reproduced by permission of the American Anthropologist 58:3, 1956. Not for further reproduction.

Nacirema culture is characterized by a highly developed market economy which has evolved in a rich natural habitat. While much of the people's time is devoted to economic pursuits, a large part of the fruits of these labors and a considerable portion of the day are spent in ritual activity. The focus of this activity is the human body, the appearance and health of which loom as a dominant concern in the ethos of the people. While such a concern is certainly not unusual, its ceremonial aspects and associated philosophy are unique.

The fundamental belief underlying the whole system appears to be that the human body is ugly and that its natural tendency is to debility and disease. Incarcerated in such a body, man's only hope is to avert these characteristics through the use of the powerful influences of ritual and ceremony. Every household has one or more shrines devoted to this purpose. The more powerful individuals in the society have several shrines in their houses and, in fact, the opulence of a house is often referred to in terms of the number of such ritual centers it possesses. Most houses are of wattle and daub construction, but the shrine rooms of the more wealthy are walled with stone. Poorer families imitate the rich by applying pottery plaques to their shrine walls.

While each family has at least one such shrine, the rituals associated with it are not family ceremonies but are private and secret. The rites are normally only discussed with children, and then only during the period when they are being initiated into these mysteries. I was able, however, to establish certainly sufficient rapport with the natives to examine these shrines and to have the rituals described to me.

The focal point of the shrine is a box or chest which is built into the wall. In this chest are kept the many charms and magical potions without which no native believes he could live. These preparations are secured from a variety of specialized practitioners. The most powerful of these are the medicine men, whose assistance must be rewarded with substantial gifts. However, the medicine men do not provide the curative potions for their clients, but decide what the ingredients should be and then write them down in an ancient and secret language. This writing is understood only by the medicine men and by the herbalists who, for another gift, provide the required charm.

The charm is not disposed of after it has served its purpose, but is placed in the charm-box of the household shrine. As these magical materials are specific for certain ills, and the real or imagined maladies of the people are many, the charm-box is usually full to overflowing. The magical packets are so numerous that people forget what their purposes were and fear to use them again. While the natives are very vague on this point, we can only assume that the idea in retaining all the old magical materials is that their presence in the charm-box, before which the body rituals are conducted, will in some way protect the worshipper.

Beneath the charm-box is a small font. Each day every member of the family, in succession, enters the shrine room, bows his head before the charm-box, mingles different sorts by holy water in the font, and proceeds with a brief rite of ablution. The holy waters are secured from the Water Temple of the community, where the priests conduct elaborate ceremonies to make the liquid ritually pure.

In the hierarchy of magical practitioners, and below the medicine men in prestige, are specialists whose designation is best translated "holy-mouth-men." The Nacirema have an almost pathological horror of and fascination with the mouth, the condition of which is believed to have a supernatural influence on all social relationships. Were it not for the rituals of the mouth they believe that their teeth would fall out, their gums bleed, their jaws shrink, their friends desert them, and their lovers reject them. They also believe that a strong relationship exists between oral and moral characteristics. For example, there is a ritual ablution of the mouth for children which is supposed to improve their moral fiber.

The daily body ritual performed by everyone includes a mouth-rite. Despite the fact that these people are so punctilious about care of the mouth, this rite involves a practice which strikes the uninitiated stranger as revolting. It was reported to me that the ritual consists of inserting a small bundle of hog hairs into the mouth, along with certain magical powders, and then removing the bundle in a highly formalized series of gestures.

In addition to the private mouth-rite, the people seek out a holy-mouth-man once or twice a year. These practitioners have an impressive set of paraphernalia, consisting of a variety of augers, awls, probes, and prods. The use of these objects in the exorcism of the evils of the mouth involves almost unbelievable ritual torture of the client. The holy-mouth-man opens the client's mouth and, using the above mentioned tools, enlarges any holes which decay may have created in the teeth. Magical materials are put into these holes. If there are no naturally occurring holes in the teeth, large sections of one or more teeth are gouged out so that the supernatural substance can be applied. In the client's view, the purpose of these ministrations is to arrest decay and to draw friends. The extremely sacred and traditional character of the rite is evident in the fact that the natives return to the holy-mouth-men year after year, despite the fact that their teeth continue to decay.

It is to be hoped that, when a thorough study of the Nacirema is made, there will be careful inquiry into the personality structure of these people. One has but to watch the gleam in the eye of a holy-mouth-man as he jabs an awl into an exposed nerve, to suspect that a certain amount of sadism is involved. If this can be established, a very interesting pattern emerges, for most of the population shows definite masochistic tendencies. It was to these that Professor Linton referred in discussing a distinctive part of the daily body ritual which is performed only by men. This part of the rite involves scraping and lacerating the surface of the face with a sharp instrument. Special women's rites are performed only four times during each lunar month, but what they lack in frequency is made up in barbarity. As part of this ceremony, women bake their heads in small ovens for about an hour. The theoretically interesting point is that what seems to be a preponderantly masochistic people have developed sadistic specialists.

The medicine men have an imposing temple, or latipsoh *in every community of any size. The more elaborate ceremonies required to treat very sick patients can only be performed at this temple. These ceremonies involve not only the thaumaturge but a permanent group of vestal maidens who move sedately about the temple chambers in distinctive costume and headdress.*

The latipsoh *ceremonies are so harsh that it is phenomenal that a fair proportion of the really sick natives who enter the temple ever recover. Small children whose indoctrination is still incomplete have been known to resist attempts to take them to the temple because "that is where you go to die." Despite this fact, sick adults are not only willing but eager to undergo the protracted ritual purification, if they can afford to do so. No matter how ill the supplicant or how grave the emergency, the guardians of many temples will not admit a client if he cannot give a rich gift to the custodian. Even after one has gained admission and survived the ceremonies, the guardians will not permit the neophyte to leave until he makes still another gift.*

The supplicant entering the temple is first stripped of all his or her clothes. In every-day life the Nacirema avoids exposure of his body and its natural functions. Bathing and excretory acts are performed only in the secrecy of the household shrine, where they are ritualized as part of the body-rites. Psychological shock results from the fact that body secrecy is suddenly lost upon entry into the latipsoh. *A man, whose own wife has never seen him in an excretory act, suddenly finds himself naked and assisted by a vestal maiden while he performs his natural functions into a sacred vessel. This sort of ceremonial treatment is necessitated by the fact that the excreta are used by a diviner to ascertain the course and nature of the client's sickness. Female clients, on the other hand, find their naked bodies are subjected to the scrutiny, manipulation, and prodding of the medicine man.*

Few supplicants in the temple are well enough to do anything but lie on their hard beds. The daily ceremonies, like the rites of the holy-mouth-man, involve discomfort and torture. With ritual precision, the vestals awaken their miserable charges each dawn and roll them about on their beds of pain while performing ablutions, in the formal movements of which the maidens are highly trained. At other times they insert magic wands in the supplicant's mouth or force him to eat substances which are supposed to be healing. From time to time the medicine men come to their clients and jab magically treated needles into their flesh. The fact that these temple ceremonies may not cure, and may even kill the neophyte in no way decreases the people's faith in the medicine men.

There remains one other kind of practitioner, known as a "listener." This witch-doctor has the power to exorcise the devils that lodge in the heads of people who have been bewitched. The Nacirema believe that parents bewitch their own children. Mothers are particularly suspected of putting a curse on children while teaching them the secret body rituals. The counter-magic of the witch-doctor is unusual in its lack of ritual. The patient simply tells the "listener" all his troubles and fears, beginning with the earliest difficulties he can remember. The memory displayed by the Nacirema in these exorcism sessions is truly remarkable. It is not uncommon for the patient to bemoan the rejection he felt upon being weaned as a babe, and a few individuals even see their troubles going back to the traumatic effect of their own birth.

In conclusion, mention must be made of certain practices which have their base in native esthetics but which depend upon the pervasive aversion to the natural body and its functions. There are ritual fasts to make fat people thin and ceremonial feasts to make thin people fat. Still other rites are used to make women's breasts larger if they are small, and smaller if they are large. General dissatisfaction with breast shape is symbolized in the fact that the ideal form is virtually outside the range of human variation. A few women afflicted with almost inhuman hypermammary development are so idolized that they make a handsome living by simply going from village to village and permitting the natives to stare at them for a fee.

Reference has already been made to the fact that excretory functions are ritualized, routinized, and relegated to secrecy. Natural reproductive functions are similarly distorted. Intercourse is taboo as a topic and scheduled as an act. Efforts are made to avoid pregnancy by the use of magical materials or by limiting intercourse to certain phases of the moon. Conception is actually very infrequent. When pregnant, women dress so as to hide their condition. Parturition takes place in secret, without friends or relatives to assist, and the majority of women do not nurse their infants.

Our review of the ritual life of the Nacirema has certainly shown them to be a magic-ridden people. It is hard to understand how they have managed to exist so long under the burdens which they have imposed upon themselves. But even such exotic customs as these take on real meaning when they are viewed with the insight provided by Malinowski when he wrote (1948:70):

> *Looking from far and above, from our high place of safety in the developed civilization, it is easy to see all the crudity and irrelevance of magic. But without its power and guidance early man could not have mastered his practical difficulties as he has done, nor could man have advanced to the higher stages of civilization.*

References Cited

Linton, Ralph. *The Study of Man.* New York: Appleton-Century, 1936.
Malinowski, Bronislaw. *Magic, Science, and Religion.* Glencoe: The Free Press, 1948.
Murdock, George P. *Social Structure.* New York: Macmillan, 1949.

DISCUSSION GUIDELINES

1. What conditions in the article tipped you off to the true identity of the Nacirema tribe?

2. Further explore and discuss Nacirema culture in relation to the following:

    a. ceremonies and rituals in a *latnem latipsoh.*

    b. witch doctor, or "listener" behavior, especially in relation to the practitioner known as an *esrun.*

3. Write a "moral" to this story.

48

Seating Arrangements in Groups

DIRECTIONS

1. Complete this tool for each session of a group therapy series. Before filling out the form the first time, duplicate sufficient copies of it for each use.

2. In the space above the chart, draw a seating diagram, viewed from above the room. Draw the walls of the room and show the arrangement of the furniture (sofas, easy chairs, straight chairs, desks, tables, etc.). Show the positions of doors and windows.

3. Identify each chair with the name of the group member occupying it.

4. Designate empty chairs with an X.

5. Use arrows to indicate how any group member alters his or her seating position during a session.

6. Use the chart to record whether members are present, absent, or late and to keep a cumulative total of absences and latenesses by each member.

7. For every group session, answer the questions that follow the chart.

SEATING DIAGRAM

Session number:

Date:

NAME OF GROUP MEMBER	PRESENT OR ABSENT	TOTAL NUMBER OF TIMES ABSENT	ON TIME OR LATE	NUMBER OF MINUTES LATE	TOTAL NUMBER OF TIMES LATE

QUESTIONS

1. What leadership activities have you undertaken about absences in specific instances? What was your rationale? What was the outcome?

2. What leadership activities have you undertaken about tardiness in specific instances? What was your rationale? What was the outcome?

3. What sense can you make of members' choices of seating?

4. How does the physical setting, including seating, influence group interaction?

49

Sociodrama Participant's Guide

A *sociodrama* is an action-oriented laboratory exercise for observing verbal and nonverbal communication and for studying and solving problems in interpersonal relationships. It focuses on the interactions between people. You can use it:

1. To learn why a nursing approach or action was ineffective.

2. To explore and try out alternative approaches.

3. To become more creative in working with clients.

4. To increase your understanding of your interpersonal dynamics.

DIRECTIONS

As a class, conduct a sociodrama session. Begin by suggesting sociodrama problems. Each problem should be:

1. One in which you were actually involved.

2. One in which you are dissatisfied with your approach or behavior.

3. One you want to explore further in order to find a more satisfactory solution.

4. One related to a specific situation with specific time limits.

Suggestions may include nurse-client problems, problems with coworkers (nursing, medical, and other personnel), problems with relatives of patients, etc.

The content of the session must be held strictly confidential. What takes place cannot be discussed outside. You are thus free to use the actual names of those who are characters in your sociodrama problem.

The instructor will help to organize and terminate the drama and lead the discussion.

1. As a group, select one of the problems suggested to focus on.

2. If you are the person whose situation was selected, request volunteer actors from the group to portray the significant persons in the situation.

163

3. Brief the actors on their roles, outside the room.

4. Return to the room, and describe the setting to the audience. Indicate what role each actor is playing. You will play yourself in the sociodrama.

5. With the other actors, reenact the situation. You may use props. Attempt to capture the mood and tone of the characters and scene rather than to reproduce the exact dialogue, ad lib while trying to maintain the mood.

6. If you are not the person whose problem is selected, and you are not chosen as an actor, you are a member of the audience. Record the proceedings (see activity 45, next). During the enactment, observe both verbal and nonverbal behaviors of the participants.

7. When the drama is terminated, relate what you saw and heard going on in the interchange, and indicate the feeling tones you detected in the nurse and the actors. You may also indicate your observations on how the relationship opened, the turning point, the "controlling" person, what the nurse's goal was and whether it was accomplished, and how the relationship ended.

8. If you were one of the actors, describe your feelings during the presentation of the problem.

9. Anyone may then suggest a different nursing approach and may volunteer to portray it. If your problem was enacted, you yourself may portray the alternative. You may continue to portray the same alternative until you become comfortable with it. Actors may reverse their roles (nurse playing client and vice versa, for example) or new cast members may be selected according to suggestions from the participants, the audience, or the instructor.

50

Sociodrama Observer's Guide

DIRECTIONS

Complete the form below as an observer in a sociodrama session (see activity 44).

Date: Session number:

Notes on Selection

Problems suggested (brief summary):

Selected Problem:

Student presenting problem:

Volunteer actor or actors:

Notes on Enactment

Verbal behavior:

Nonverbal behavior:

Feeling tones:

Opening of relationship:

Controlling person:

Turning point:

Subject's goals and extent of accomplishment:

Other significant observations:

Closing of relationship:

Notes on Discussion

Issues during discussion (specify initiator of issue):

Nursing alternatives offered:

Nursing alternative selected:

Comments:

51

Group Coleader's Inventory

This tool is designed to help you establish and maintain an egalitarian coleading relationship.

DIRECTIONS

Before beginning a group therapy experience with a coleader, complete tasks 1 through 5. Your coleader should do the same.

1. In the space below, write approximately 100 words explaining your concept of how group therapy helps people. Refer to the theorists and theories that guide your work.

2. List at least ten things that you expect to happen in the group you will be coleading. Identify the very *worst*, and the very *best* things that could happen.

EXPECTATIONS

BEST POSSIBILITY	WORST POSSIBILITY

3. Complete the following statements about your typical responses in therapeutic work with clients:

When beginning the relationship, I usually

When someone talks too much, I usually

When a client is silent, I usually

When someone cries, I usually

When someone comes late, I usually

When people are excessively polite and unwilling to confront each other, I usually

When there is conflict in a group, I usually

When one individual is verbally attacked, I usually

If there is physical violence, I usually

When clients discuss sexual feelings about others, or about me, I usually

My "favorite" interventions are

My typical intervention "rhythm" (fast/slow) is

My style is characteristically more (nurturing/confronting)

The thing that makes me most uncomfortable in groups is

4.   Complete the information below on your past group experiences

APPROXIMATE DATES	DURATION	TYPE OF GROUP	MY ROLE

5. List your scores from self-assessment instruments, such as activities 1, 6, 7, 9, 13, 16, and 18 of this workbook, that have helped you understand yourself better. Comment on what these data mean in terms of an egalitarian coleader relationship.

Exchange the above responses with your coleader. Share your reactions to the exchange of information and elaborate for each other where necessary.

Together complete tasks 6 through 13.

6. Do activity 47, "Coleader Encounter," next in this workbook.

7. State some of your coleader behavior patterns, and indicate the behaviors your coleader might see as idiosyncratic.

8. Describe the personal growth efforts that you are making right now. Indicate what personal growth goals you anticipate working on during this group experience.

9. Note issues that have arisen in your past work with other coleaders.

10. Discuss your reactions to the makeup of the group, its size, and any other special considerations.

11. Set up operating norms and a coleader contract:

    a. Where will you each sit in the group meetings?

    b. Who will begin and end each session?

    c. How will lateness and absence be handled?

    d. How much "there-and-then" discussion will be allowed, and how do you define "here-and-now"?

    e. Will you make theory inputs? If so, how?

    f. What will you do about group members' requests for contacts outside the group?

12. Discuss your anticipated coleading style:

    a. Where, when, and how will you deal with issues between the two of you?

    b. Can you agree to disagree?

    c. Will you encourage or discourage conflict?

    d. How much of your behavior will be role determined, and how much will be personal and individual?

    e. Is it possible for you to use each other s energy—that is, can one of you be "out" while the other is "in"?

    f. How will you establish and maintain growth-producing norms?

    g. What is nonnegotiable for each of you as coleader?

13. Discuss your ethics:

    a. What responsibilities do you each have after the group experience is over? Are you responsible for referral?

    b. What responsibilities do you have for screening?

    c. Are you adequately qualified? How have you communicated your qualifications to the group?

    d. What are your standards with regard to confidentiality?

After each group session, complete tasks 14 through 16.

14. Analyze the group:

    a. On a ten-point scale, how did things go in this meeting?

    b. What is happening in the group?

    c. Is anyone "hurting"?

    d. What are the themes?

    e. Which group dynamics are operative?

15. Solicit feedback from each other by asking:

    a. What did I do that was effective?

    b. What did I do that was ineffective?

    c. How am I working as a coleader?

    d. What else would you like from me that I'm not giving?

16. Consider renegotiating the coleadership contract:

    a. Is there anything that you need to renegotiate?

    b. How are you feeling about each other?

    c. What is each of you going to do in the next group meeting?

After the final group session, complete task 17.

17. Terminate the coleading relationship:

    a. Discuss the extent to which your personal goals were achieved.

    b. Discuss under what conditions you would work together again.

    c. Discuss your personal and professional learning from this experience.

    d. Solicit ideas for your continued personal growth.

    e. Solicit ideas about improving your group-leading competence.

52

Coleader Encounter

When you communicate with another person, your responses are formed by your perceptions of that person. In other words, when you talk to another, you are actually talking to an image you have of that person. Your image may not be the same as the image the person has of himself or herself.

In order to establish a mutual world with another, you need to find out about the "real" other person, to obtain an accurate picture of that person's self-image. What questions should you ask in order to obtain an accurate perception? This exercise is designed to help you find out.

DIRECTIONS

Below list ten questions your coleader should ask in order to know the "real" you. Exchange lists with your coleader. You have thirty minutes in which to interview each other using the questions your coleader has provided to achieve the most self-disclosure. Write out your coleader's answers to her or his ten questions. Your coleader will write down your answers to your questions. Discuss your answers with one another.

1.

2.

3.

4.

5.

6.

7.

8.

9.

10.

53

Guide to Interaction Process Analysis

In order to learn the function of therapeutic intervention, the process of a therapeutic nurse-client relationship, you must be able to study and review with objectivity the components of this process. As the responsible individual in the interaction, you must review both verbal and nonverbal components for their potential meaning. They may be expressing problems or attempts at resolving problems. The tool used for this review is the *interaction process analysis*. An IPA is a verbatim and progressive recording of the verbal and nonverbal interactions between client and nurse within a given period of time. It consists of:

1. A summary of the circumstances associated with the recorded interaction.

2. An accurate and objective recording of the verbal and behavioral communication between client and nurse within the period. It may describe nonverbal communication alone, if conversation does not occur. If conversation does occur, the IPA must both record the words and describe accompanying nonverbal communication by each participant in the interaction. Nonverbal behavior is described in parentheses. Exchanges must be recorded in proper sequence, to indicate the direction of the communication.

3. For each significant communication (verbal or nonverbal), a statement in the nurse- or the client-centered analysis (or both) that specifies the following:

   a. An analysis or interpretation of the possible meaning of the communication,

   b. Identification of the nurse's own emotions and the possible intent of the nurse's communication, whether conscious or unconscious,

   c. Perceptions of the emotions expressed by the client and the intent of the client's communication, whether conscious or unconscious,

   d. Evaluation of the effectiveness of the nurse's approach, based on the above data,

   e. Suggestions of nursing alternatives in order of their usefulness.

DIRECTIONS

Prepare an interaction process analysis for each of several sessions with your client. Before filling out the form the first time, duplicate sufficient copies of it for each use.

INTERACTION PROCESS ANALYSIS

Circumstances

Description of environmental setting:

Feeling tone

  Nurse's:

  Client's:

  Unit milieu:

Description of client:

Significant data prior to interaction:

Goals

  Nurse-centered:

Client-centered:

Interaction Process Analysis

INTERACTION (Verbal and Nonverbal)	NURSE-CENTERED ANALYSIS	CLIENT-CENTERED ANALYSIS

INTERACTION (VERBAL AND NONVERBAL)	NURSE-CENTERED ANALYSIS	CLIENT-CENTERED ANALYSIS

Summary

Themes perceived in interaction:

Evaluation in terms of goals
  Nurse-centered goals:

  Client-centered goals:

References to theory (articles or books read as preparation for IPA):

54

Analyzing a Crisis Call

DIRECTIONS

Analyze the following verbatim recording of a call taken by a nurse at a crisis intervention center. In making your analysis, refer to activity 50, "Guide to Interaction Process Analysis." The conversation is presented in the IPA format.

Interaction Process Analysis

INTERACTION (VERBAL AND NONVERBAL)	NURSE-CENTERED ANALYSIS	CLIENT-CENTERED ANALYSIS
Nurse: Can I help you?		
Caller: Yes, you may (crying).		
Nurse: You sound pretty upset. What seems to be the problem?		
Caller: I don't know. It's just too much to go on.		
Nurse: What's going on now that seems like too much?		
Caller: My mother just died.		
Nurse: Your mother just died?		
Caller: Yes.		
Nurse: When was that?		

INTERACTION (VERBAL AND NONVERBAL)	NURSE-CENTERED ANALYSIS	CLIENT-CENTERED ANALYSIS
Caller (crying): Excuse me. About a week ago.		
Nurse: Wow—that's pretty upsetting, isn't it?		
Caller: I just can't take any more bad things happening to me (crying).		
Nurse: What else has been happening to you?		
Caller: All kinds of problems.		
Nurse: Like what?		
Caller: Boys and parties and all sorts of stuff. (Cries.) I don't know what to do.		
Nurse: You're feeling really low now, aren't you?		
Caller: Pardon?		
Nurse: You're feeling really low now.		
Caller: Yes.		
Nurse: How do you feel about your mother's death?		
Caller: Alone. My father doesn't want me.		
Nurse: What?		
Caller: My father doesn't want me.		
Nurse: Where are you going to end up then?		

INTERACTION (VERBAL AND NONVERBAL)	NURSE-CENTERED ANALYSIS	CLIENT-CENTERED ANALYSIS
Caller: I don't know.		
Nurse: Your father doesn't want you?		
Caller: No.		
Nurse: How do you know?		
Caller: He said so.		
Nurse: Can you tell me your name?		
Caller: No.		
Nurse: Just your first name?		
Caller: No.		
Nurse: Okay. Who are you staying with now?		
Caller: My aunt.		
Nurse: So your aunt wants you.		
Caller: Yes—I guess so.		
Nurse: How long have you been staying with her?		
Caller: About a couple of days.		
Nurse: So you haven't stayed with your father in a few days, is that it?		
Caller: Yes.		
Nurse: That's . . . that's pretty . . . that's pretty damn upsetting.		

INTERACTION (VERBAL AND NONVERBAL)	NURSE-CENTERED ANALYSIS	CLIENT-CENTERED ANALYSIS
Caller: It is; it sure is.		
Nurse: To know that your father doesn't want you. I don't blame you for crying about that.		
Caller: What?		
Nurse: I said I don't blame you for crying about that.		
Caller: I just don't know what to do, I can't stand it.		
Nurse: How long have you been feeling like this?		
Caller: Oh, for a long time.		
Nurse: Do you have any other brothers and sisters?		
Caller: No.		
Nurse: You're the only child?		
Caller: Yes.		
Nurse: Do you know why he doesn't want you?		
Caller: No. (crying).		
Nurse: He didn't tell you?		
Caller: No. He just didn't give me any reason. He wants to go his own way (crying).		
Nurse: That's . . . that's hurt your feelings.		
Caller: Yes.		

INTERACTION (VERBAL AND NONVERBAL)	NURSE-CENTERED ANALYSIS	CLIENT-CENTERED ANALYSIS
Nurse: What is he doing now? Caller: I don't know. Nurse: You haven't heard from him? Caller: No. Nurse: In how long? Caller: In a very long time . . . . (Hangs up.)		

55

Analyzing an Individual Session

DIRECTIONS

Analyze the following verbatim recording of a second session with a client in individual relationship therapy. In making your analysis, refer to activity 50, "Guide to Interaction Process Analysis."

The client, Jennie, is a twenty-six-year-old woman who lives with her five-year-old daughter. Scott, her husband, moved out of the house last month. Jennie was briefly hospitalized in a psychiatric unit three years ago with a diagnosis of "obsessive-compulsive reaction."

Interaction Process Analysis

INTERACTION (VERBAL AND NONVERBAL)	NURSE-CENTERED ANALYSIS	CLIENT-CENTERED ANALYSIS
(Jennie arrives fifteen minutes late.) Nurse: Hi, Jennie. Jennie: Hi. The cab was a little late. Nurse: You took a cab? Jennie: Yeah. It's freezing out and I knew that . . . I . . . didn't feel like walking up (laugh), plus I . . . I was . . . um . . . (quietly) getting ready at the last minute, anyway.		

INTERACTION (VERBAL AND NONVERBAL)	NURSE-CENTERED ANALYSIS	CLIENT-CENTERED ANALYSIS
Nurse: Ah hum. Sometimes you have trouble getting going?		
Jennie: Yes!		
(Silence.)		
Nurse: So how are things going?		
Jennie: Um . . . last night . . . not so well.		
Nurse: Not so well?		
Jennie: Oh . . . (low voice) I don't know, I guess. It happened after I ate dinner. I just, I don't know if it's the low blood sugar or nerves or what. I mean it *acts* like low blood sugar.		
Nurse: How's that? You mentioned this before—with low blood sugar you have certain symptoms, and you feel like you know when it's happening. How does it feel?		
Jennie: Well . . . like, first, I guess, first I notice that my thinking was getting worse. And, like, it was harder to *think* and harder to concentrate. And, like, I never realized . . . I thought some of that business was just emotions and being upset, and then, after reading this book I have on low blood sugar, it explains that . . . like, if your blood sugar is low, well it's low for your whole body, so		

INTERACTION (VERBAL AND NONVERBAL)	NURSE-CENTERED ANALYSIS	CLIENT-CENTERED ANALYSIS
your brain is only half nourished, like, with sugar—(quietly) so it's just not going to work as well. So . . . you know . . . it's probably that. But I guess emotions can trigger off stuff like that, too. But, then, food has something to do with it, cause they put you on a special diet, you know, and . . . but then . . . once your blood sugar gets low, you can get . . . like, I started to get real irritable and feeling depressed and . . . um . . . then my ears get real sensitive to noise—like the kids were playing . . . and they weren't that loud, I'm sure . . . ah . . . but it started pounding in my ears, and then I had to leave the room, it hurt so bad. Nurse: Um hum. Jennie: But all the symptoms were of low blood sugar. The doctor doesn't know what's causing it, you know . . . ah . . . I guess a lot of times they don't know, and then sometimes they can find out? Nurse: Yes, I would think the physical and emotional could both be contributing, and this may be an area we'll want to sort out more clearly—perhaps have some physical work done soon. I wonder if we could look at the emotional question for a time here, though . . . I'm wondering, Jennie, when did all these feelings start yesterday? What time of day was it?		

INTERACTION (VERBAL AND NONVERBAL)	NURSE-CENTERED ANALYSIS	CLIENT-CENTERED ANALYSIS
Jennie: Ah, it was after supper.		
Nurse: And before that time you were feeling—how?		
Jennie: Ah, I wasn't real good, I was . . . um . . . I wasn't all that irritable or anything, but I was having trouble concentrating and thinking, which I have most all the time.		
Nurse: Ah huh.		
Jennie: It's just like . . . (surprised) Well, the day before I was thinking good! I was thinking more clearly.		
Nurse: Were you anticipating something happening?		
Jennie: Well, Scott was supposed to call that night, that's the only thing I can think of that would make me a little nervous. But actually I didn't really want to see him 'cause I wasn't thinking that clearly. The night before I was thinking good and I thought I *could talk* to him. But then last night—yesterday—I wasn't thinking all that well . . . . I don't think I slept good the night before . . . um . . . but (quietly) I don't know exactly why I wasn't sleeping good, whether it was that, I don't know.		
Nurse: Jennie, I'm wondering— what feelings you were having last night. Was it a fearful feeling?		

INTERACTION (VERBAL AND NONVERBAL)	NURSE-CENTERED ANALYSIS	CLIENT-CENTERED ANALYSIS
Jennie: Um . . . (long pause). No. I had those . . . um, not really. I don't think it was. Maybe it was a little bit . . . um . . . well, maybe because of it I felt afraid that . . . er . . . because (slower, very quiet) I don't like to be sick like that. Nurse: Ah huh? Jennie: But I . . . I don't really know . . . . I wouldn't say it was really *fear*, but it . . . bothered me that I felt like that. But, but I have had fear at other times . . . like . . . going to sleep and . . . well, I don't know if it's fear or rejection or what—you know, but . . . thinking about Scott . . . (eyes tearing) . . . I don't really know if it's fear. Nurse: Ah huh. What *does* it feel like? (Silence.) Jennie: I guess . . . (silence, tearing, looking down into lap as though to attempt to compose herself). Nurse: You look so sad to me. Are you thinking about Scott and what's happening between you, when you speak of rejection? Jennie (crying): I don't think I can talk about that (looking very sad, tears coming down her cheeks but with no sobbing —very controlled crying).		

INTERACTION (VERBAL AND NONVERBAL)	NURSE-CENTERED ANALYSIS	CLIENT-CENTERED ANALYSIS
Nurse: It's really hard for you to talk about it, I see. (Pause.) Nurse: Are you able to cry about it sometimes? Jennie (softly): Yeah, at home I can. Nurse: How is it for you? Jennie (softly): I don't know . . . I guess it . . . it helps sometimes. (Pause.) A lot of times when he was there though, I couldn't. Nurse: When he was there you couldn't cry? Jennie (continues quietly): Yeah, because he never . . . always . . . I don't know . . . he just never liked to see me cry. He'd leave the room or something, or . . . or I'd go in the bedroom . . . . He'd just never like to see me cry. Or if he'd see me . . . if I was crying . . . during the nervous breakdown he'd . . . he'd just, um, he'd just shake his head and walk away. Nurse: You had to keep your crying—and feelings—from him. He acted as though your way of trying to communicate feelings was a sign of . . . weakness? Jennie: Yes! And he'd act like		

INTERACTION (VERBAL AND NONVERBAL)	NURSE-CENTERED ANALYSIS	CLIENT-CENTERED ANALYSIS
it was just a sign of a breakdown.		
Nurse: That must have been so painful, to have to keep so many feelings inside. . . . What things were you feeling that were making you sad?		
Jennie: What I was going through . . . what I was going through during the nervous breakdown and . . . and also the fact that . . . (long pause) that he wasn't there to reassure me or anything (voice fragile).		
Nurse: That you were alone in this.		
Jennie: Yes. And instead of reassuring me he just went the other way . . . started to shake his head at me. Put me down for it. He . . . I don't think he did that right at the beginning but he . . . (quietly) he finally did it.		
Nurse: So . . . you were holding your feelings in, because they were making it hard on him?		
Jenning (cuts in): Maybe. Because, I guess, it's because, not because it was . . . hard on him . . . it's because whenever I did it . . . he'd look down on me, you know.		
Nurse: What do you think he was thinking? Looking down on you.		
Jennie: That I was . . .		

INTERACTION (VERBAL AND NONVERBAL)	NURSE-CENTERED ANALYSIS	CLIENT-CENTERED ANALYSIS
incapable and . . . weak and not happy and . . . Nurse: Because you were crying? Jennie: Well, not just the crying, it was like he'd see me . . . into the nervous . . . thing of the nervous breakdown, you know, where I seem to be compelled to wash my hands, something like that . . . because, I had fears and I wasn't thinking very . . . I don't know . . . it was all . . . it was all the fears. Nurse: Um hum. Jennie: But I never realized it when I was having a nervous breakdown, but, everything that, um, everything . . . the four main things that I had with the nervous breakdown were. . . . Um . . . I think (looking at tape recorder), I think it's bothering me to have that on. Nurse: Oh. Well, maybe it's best that we talk about it, if you feel that it's difficult. Are there things you wanted to say that you're hesitating? Jennie: Well. What were we talking about? Nurse: You were about to tell me that there were four things . . . about the nervous breakdown.		

INTERACTION (VERBAL AND NONVERBAL)	NURSE-CENTERED ANALYSIS	CLIENT-CENTERED ANALYSIS
Jennie: Oh yeah, after I found out—like a couple of years later—that I had low blood sugar, um, after reading some of the things the doctor gave me and then . . . um, some of the . . . a book I had on it . . . those four things were . . . well, they could be symptoms of other things but they're also symptoms of low blood sugar. . . . And the doctor never tested me for low blood sugar.		
Nurse: When you had the nervous breakdown?		
Jennie: Yeah, they never did.		
Nurse: Are you wondering now, if, when you had the breakdown, if it could have been caused by the low blood sugar—if, because there wasn't a test done at that time, . . .		
Jennie: Wait, I'm lost at the beginning.		
Nurse: Are you thinking now that the breakdown might have been caused by low blood sugar?		
Jennie: I'm thinking it could have been.		
Nurse: That's something you're questioning. . . . Um, I don't . . . I can't give you an answer for that, but I think what you're going . . .		
Jennie (cuts in): You know		

INTERACTION (VERBAL AND NONVERBAL)	NURSE-CENTERED ANALYSIS	CLIENT-CENTERED ANALYSIS
(laugh), that tape recorder bothers me. Nurse: Okay. Let's turn it off. (Turns off tape.) (In the remainder of the session, Jennie related her fears of being seen as "crazy" and of feeling "crazy." She discussed her mother's long history of "crazy" behavior. Jennie fears a sick label for herself.)		

56

Analyzing a Group Session

DIRECTIONS

Analyze the following verbatim recording of a session of an ongoing outpatient psychotherapy group led by cotherapists. In making your analysis, refer to activity 50, "Guide to Interaction Process Analysis."

The group members are:

Janeen, thirty-three-year-old housewife, with three children, ages four, two and a half, and sixteen months. She has held several low-paying, low-status jobs during her married years. She expresses herself by complete submissiveness, and is fearful of losing control of the intense rage she feels. Janeen has a low self-concept and low self-esteem and cries frequently. She wants to find herself but fears that in doing so she may have to make some decisions regarding her marital situation. Although Janeen describes her marriage as intolerable, she states she loves her husband and wants to preserve the marriage. She has made one suicide attempt.

Linda, thirty-five-year-old housewife, with three children, ages nine, six, and four. Linda has never worked outside the home. She has often threatened her alcoholic husband with separation but is unable to carry through. She reacts to multiple humiliations with either passivity or rage. Linda is terrified to live alone, sure that she cannot support herself and the children. She is unaware of her legal rights regarding alimony and property division. She has a poor self-concept and low self-esteem and wants to develop confidence in herself.

Mary Ann, fifty-two-year-old widow, with four married children and one sixteen-year-old daughter. This daughter was turned away from the home because she was unmanageable. Mary Ann is depressed, feels worthless, and has little hope that things will ever change. At thirty-five years of age she suffered a heart attack and was told by her physician that she was disabled. Mary Ann is submissive in all problem situations, describing herself as a doormat. She often feels suicidal but has not made an attempt.

Lisa, twenty-two-year-old housewife, who holds a full-time job as a graphic artist. Lisa lived with her husband for four years before they married. She professes to adhere to modern views on life, but finds herself powerless within the confines of her marriage. Lisa admits to severe marital difficulties but is unable to consider living alone. She is depressed and thinks of suicide but has not made any attempts. Lisa feels isolated and alienated, believing that others will not understand her. Her feeling of self-worth is low.

Nancy, the fifth member of the group, who did not attend the session or call to say that she wouldn't be able to come.

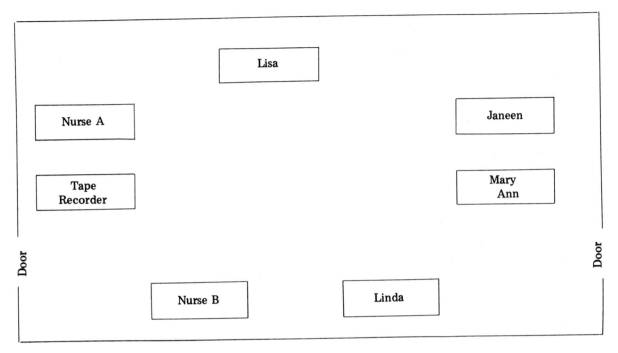

Figure 2. Seating chart, group therapy session 2

Interaction Process Analysis

INTERACTION (VERBAL AND NONVERBAL)	NURSE-CENTERED ANALYSIS	CLIENT-CENTERED ANALYSIS
Mary Ann: I've been doing a lot of thinking about this group this past week. Could you tell me what this group is supposed to do for you anyway?		
Nurse B: I wonder if anyone might want to help Mary Ann out with that?		
Janeen: I think it's been too easy for us to dwell only on ourselves. After a while, I begin to think I'm the only one that has any problems. Being in this		

INTERACTION (VERBAL AND NONVERBAL)	NURSE-CENTERED ANALYSIS	CLIENT-CENTERED ANALYSIS
group is showing me that I'm not the only one with a problem. (Others nod in agreement.) Linda: Maybe it's easier to say things here that maybe you wouldn't say anywhere else. Lisa: It's been important for me to see that other people can have problems. I agree that it's pretty easy to sit and feel sorry for yourself . . . as if nobody can be as miserable as you. Nurse B: A group like this can give people an opportunity to look at each other and look at themselves in an open and honest way. It could give you a better understanding of your relationships with other people. Nurse A: Yes. It can also be a safe place to say things and try different ways of handling problems. Mary Ann: I have something I'd like to try out on the group. My sister-in-law sent me an invitation to a luncheon. She's the sort of person who knows everybody, and everything has to be the best. I am not going to go. (There is a little flurry of activity, and several people speak in unison.) Lisa: I don't think you should		

INTERACTION (VERBAL AND NONVERBAL)	NURSE-CENTERED ANALYSIS	CLIENT-CENTERED ANALYSIS
stay away just because they have more than you do. Just because they have more money than you doesn't mean they are better than you. I think you should go. You might have a good time.		
Janeen: Having money doesn't mean much. I know a man who has a lot of money and is as nice as anyone could want. But then, there is another man who has a lot of money. He is an executive and has everything anyone could want. He is as nasty as can be. So, I don't think it makes any difference how much money anyone has. You're just as good as they are. I think you should go, too.		
Linda: Sure you should go. You can't just sit home and feel sorry for yourself. Just go. After you're there for a while, I bet you'll forget about it and have a good time.		
Mary Ann: But the money doesn't bother me. I don't think they are better than me. It's something else and I don't know what it is. Guilt I guess. I always feel guilty. Maybe they'll reject me.		
(Again the members try to give her support and encouragement. The group is talking spontaneously and the atmosphere is one of support and good feelings for each other.)		

INTERACTION (VERBAL AND NONVERBAL)	NURSE-CENTERED ANALYSIS	CLIENT-CENTERED ANALYSIS
Janeen (to Mary Ann): You know, I've been thinking about you this week. You are in a position to be able to do anything you want to. With no husband or kids to take care of, you . . . you could even go back to school, or get a job.		
Mary Ann: I've worked before. I worked for years at Community Hospital, but I don't know if I could do it physically.		
Lisa: They have some really interesting courses at the university that you could look into.		
Mary Ann: I don't know. Maybe I can't do it. What if I can't make it?		
Linda: You can always start easy. Look into the credit-free programs at the university. They cost very little money, and, if you are worried about failing or not doing well, they won't be marking you.		
Mary Ann: I don't know. It just seems so hard to do. Tell me, how do you go about it? How do you change your life?		
Linda: You just do it! You do it one step at a time.		
Janeen: No one else can do it for you. We can only give you suggestions, but you have to do it.		

INTERACTION (VERBAL AND NONVERBAL)	NURSE-CENTERED ANALYSIS	CLIENT-CENTERED ANALYSIS
(Lisa nods in agreement.)		
(The group gradually became more silent as Mary Ann continued to block their suggestions. She then dominated the session with stories of her failure as a mother—her youngest son and daughter have been in a lot of trouble. She went on to discuss the many severe beatings her youngest daughter had at the hands of other family members.)		
Mary Ann: I didn't hit her. I never stopped them either. I just stood by and let them beat her. Of course at the time I was very angry too. Was I wrong?		
(Silence.)		
Nurse B: I wonder if the group might try to answer Mary Ann.		
Linda: Well, I think you were wrong. Maybe you were not involved, but you let it go on.		
(Mary Ann continued to be verbally active, while the other members became more and more silent.		
Nurse A: I notice how different this meeting is from the last meeting. I'm wondering what you think the difference might be. . . . These silences seem very uncomfortable.		
(Silence.)		

INTERACTION (VERBAL AND NONVERBAL)	*NURSE-CENTERED ANALYSIS*	*CLIENT-CENTERED ANALYSIS*
Nurse B: Mary Ann seems to be blocking all your suggestions for help. That must be frustrating for the person who is trying to help. (Silence.) (Mary Ann began talking again about being afraid to go out socially. She believes people are talking about her because of all the "bad things" her children have done—their trouble with the law.) Linda (emphatically): Well, I think that's very unreasonable. My husband is a heavy drinker and has done many things to embarrass me, but I no longer assume any responsibility for his actions. (An extremely long silence—four or five minutes.) Janeen: I don't want to take up too much time talking about myself, but there is one thing I would like to say. I saw my father a few weeks ago for the first time in about thirteen years. It was really nice. Better than it's ever been. He's been in Florida. He brought me frozen shrimp and lobster, and they were just great. He said, "The one thing I really feel bad about is the fact that your mother never loved you." So that's all I am going to say. (Another silence. Mary Ann		

INTERACTION (VERBAL AND NONVERBAL)	NURSE-CENTERED ANALYSIS	CLIENT-CENTERED ANALYSIS
occasionally began talking but eventually became silent. This silence also lasted for four or five minutes. Janeen was tearful and appeared angry and/or sad.)		
Nurse A: There is definitely something going on here, even though it's silent. As I look around, I can see some sad faces, and I see some angry faces.		
Mary Ann: Maybe we need some humor around here. Has anyone heard about the traveling salesman?		
Linda: No, Mary Ann. What is it?		
Mary Ann: I guess I forgot it.		
Janeen: Knock, knock!		
Mary Ann: Who's there?		
Janeen: Sarah.		
Mary Ann: Sarah, who?		
Janeen: Sarah Doctor in the house?		
(Polite laughs around the room. Again the group reverted to silence. The tension seemed to mount, and finally Janeen stood up.)		
Janeen (briskly): Children are sweet and innocent things. I am going home. (She got her hat and coat and left.)		

INTERACTION (VERBAL AND NONVERBAL)	NURSE-CENTERED ANALYSIS	CLIENT-CENTERED ANALYSIS
Nurse B: I'm feeling surprised that Janeen would leave without explaining to us why she felt she needed to go. I wonder how everyone is feeling about this?		
Lisa: I had a feeling that she didn't want to be here in the first place.		
Mary Ann: I just have this feeling that somehow I chased her away. I feel responsible.		
Nurse A: When a member leaves or is missing, it affects the whole group.		
Linda: I think that the girl who is not here (referring to Nancy) is different though. She never said anything to us. We didn't know anything about her.		
Mary Ann: I think Janeen left because she told us too much about herself last week. I think she felt too uncomfortable with us.		
Nurse B: Mary Ann, you have told us a great deal about yourself tonight.		
Mary Ann: Well, I'll be here next week. I gave you my commitment for the next twelve weeks, and I'll be here.		
Lisa: You know, I've been thinking whether this group is right for me or not. I heard there is a group of younger		

INTERACTION (VERBAL AND NONVERBAL)	NURSE-CENTERED ANALYSIS	CLIENT-CENTERED ANALYSIS
people here, but then . . . I don't know whether that would be right either. It doesn't seem as if my problems have anything in common with any of you women. My life-style is very different.		
Mary Ann: Maybe I'm older than you, but what makes you think you won't be in the same position as I am when you are my age? We're all the same.		
Lisa: Well, for one thing, I won't have six kids.		
Mary Ann: Do you think I'm going to treat you like a mother would?		
Lisa: You already have.		
Mary Ann: What do you mean? How?		
Lisa: For one thing, you were very upset when you talked about your daughter smoking pot. I smoke pot, and I don't think I'm terrible.		
(Both Mary Ann and Linda laugh loudly.)		
Linda: I hate to disillusion you but I've smoked pot lots of times before.		
Lisa (clearly shocked): But I mean on a regular basis.		
Linda: The only reason I don't smoke more often is that I just		

INTERACTION (VERBAL AND NONVERBAL)	NURSE-CENTERED ANALYSIS	CLIENT-CENTERED ANALYSIS
don't like it. It's not that big of a deal, you know. (The group paused, seeming to consider what had just occurred.) Nurse A: We only have about five minutes left. Maybe we could spend the time talking about what happened tonight and how you feel about it. Lisa: I know things are a little better for me, but I don't know what I can do about my mother-in-law. I think she is my biggest problem now. (Lisa then goes into specific detail on how she has been mistreated by her mother-in-law and made to be a pawn in the battle between mother and son.) Nurse B: So, it seems then, that, although the problems one has may be different from someone else's, the pain they cause isn't. Nurse A: Maybe the way that people respond to their problems might be important in learning how to make things easier. The problems may be different but feelings are shared by everyone. (Again a silence, but the tension that was present earlier was absent.)		

INTERACTION (VERBAL AND NONVERBAL)	NURSE-CENTERED ANALYSIS	CLIENT-CENTERED ANALYSIS
Nurse B: I want to remind you all that membership in the group is open, and there may be new members next week. (At this point, people began to leave the room.)		

57

Analyzing Marital Couple Interaction

DIRECTIONS

Analyze the following verbatim recording of a second session with a couple in marital therapy. In making your analysis, refer to activity 50, "Guide to Interaction Process Analysis."

Tom and Karen have been married for twelve years. Karen had telephoned the mental health agency because of "serious marital problems" that needed to be talked about. They have an eleven-year-old son, Mark, but did not wish to include him in sessions at this time due to the "urgent" and "adult" nature of the problems.

Tom had a medical history of a spontaneous pneumothorax four years ago and has suffered terrible coughing spasms since then. The episode altered his view on life toward "getting all the enjoyment I can—I could probably drop dead any time!"

During the week following the first therapy session, Karen called saying that they had again talked and that Tom had "let it all out." He told her he had an extramarital relationship of two years' standing. On the phone with Karen the nurse suggested the three of them talk about this at the next session.

INTERACTION (VERBAL AND NONVERBAL)	NURSE-CENTERED ANALYSIS	CLIENT-CENTERED ANALYSIS
Nurse: Let's see . . . I talked with you, Karen, on Thursday.		
Karen: Yes, Thursday night.		
(Silence.)		
Nurse: Karen let me know, Tom, that you and she had had a further conversation the night after our first meeting.		

INTERACTION (VERBAL AND NONVERBAL)	NURSE-CENTERED ANALYSIS	CLIENT-CENTERED ANALYSIS
Tom: Um hum.		
Nurse: . . . and that you had shared with her the fact that you have been involved with another woman. Karen told me of this briefly, over the phone. I asked her if she could talk about it here, instead, as I want our work together to take place when we're all here, so that we all have the same base to work from.		
Tom: Yes, she told me she had talked with you. (Monotone, low voice. Contrasts with his "cocky" manner the week before.)		
(Silence.)		
Nurse: Maybe there are things either of you would like to share here		
Karen: Why don't you start? (Looks to Tom.)		
Tom: You start—go ahead.		
(Pause.)		
Tom: I don't know what to say. You go ahead.		
Nurse: Kind of hard to talk about things?		
Karen: Well, I explained to her (looking at Tom) about your friend . . .		
Tom: Um hum.		

INTERACTION (VERBAL AND NONVERBAL)	NURSE-CENTERED ANALYSIS	CLIENT-CENTERED ANALYSIS
Karen: . . . and I asked her if she felt we should continue with this. And . . . ah . . . she said . . . we should . . . and that . . . whatever happens we'd have to prepare Mark for this.		
Tom: Um hum.		
Karen: 'Cause he's part of this family.		
Tom: Right.		
Karen: So . . . that's that.		
(Silence.)		
Nurse: I guess I'm thinking— not only to prepare Mark, but for yourselves too—it may be useful to talk more on what you have begun. I'm thinking that sometimes moves are made impulsively. It may be that you aren't looking to a separation, for instance . . . or that you may want time to think about it. How is it for you?		
Tom: Right! . . . Ah, I would like time to think this over. To see if it's what I really want to do. . . . Ah . . . This friend of mine, I . . . I don't expect to marry . . . at least I don't think so, not right away. . . . It's just that . . . well . . . we get along together real well. Of course we don't live together. I suppose if we did maybe we'd find fault in one another . . . like when, you know, when you're married to someone!		

INTERACTION (VERBAL AND NONVERBAL)	NURSE-CENTERED ANALYSIS	CLIENT-CENTERED ANALYSIS
Nurse: Things about being married make it somewhat different?		
Tom: Yeah . . . yeah. Just like, well, after we got married we found out things about one another that . . . while they looked real rosy before we got married . . . then it's not quite so good afterwards.		
Nurse: How about that, Karen, how's it been for you?		
Karen: Well, you can't just have all sweetness and light when you're married. Somebody's got to take care of things. . . . Things do change . . .		
Tom (interrupts): But . . . ah . . . rather than just move out tomorrow . . . I would like some time to think about it and . . . if I do move out . . . ah . . . we would have to come to an amicable agreement or understanding. So that neither one of us gets taken to the dry cleaners . . . or . . . gets hurt. But . . . it's something that should take time and consideration to think about.		
Nurse: Are you asking Karen for some time to think things through?		
Tom: Yeah.		
Nurse (gestures toward Karen): Can you ask her directly?		

INTERACTION (VERBAL AND NONVERBAL)	NURSE-CENTERED ANALYSIS	CLIENT-CENTERED ANALYSIS
Tom: Oh . . . yeah. . . . I . . . I wish we . . . could think about this . . . before making any decisions. . . . (Pause.) Maybe it's just the idea that I would like my freedom, so that I can do as I please without hurting her.		
Nurse: Who?		
Tom: Oh . . . hurting you (to Karen) or Mark or . . . having a guilt complex about it. I just . . . if I want to . . . stay out late or go someplace . . . I don't want to have to be responsible to her . . . (low voice) to anyone but myself.		
Karen: (Loud coughing.)		
Nurse (looking to Karen): You'd like to respond to Tom?		
Karen (speaking rapidly): You mean when he first told me about this? (Seems to be attempting to control anger.)		
Nurse: Or now?		
Karen: Well . . . I feel if that's what he wants he should have it! If he wants his freedom— and feels that there isn't enough happiness here—I feel that's due him. Just as it's due me. I mean it wouldn't be fair for me to take it away from him, and it wouldn't be fair for him to take it away from me.		

INTERACTION (VERBAL AND NONVERBAL)	NURSE-CENTERED ANALYSIS	CLIENT-CENTERED ANALYSIS
Nurse: I'm puzzled. Go on with that a bit in terms of how it is for you. Karen: Well . . . I've had my suspicions . . . and I felt that there would come a time when he would just . . . tell me. And I felt . . . well, why . . . push the issue. . . . When the time is right, he'll just . . . cough it up! (Blows smoke in his direction.) (The rest of the time was spent planning future sessions. The three agreed to focus on getting in touch with the anger and hurt each partner had experienced.)		

58

Analyzing Family Interaction

DIRECTIONS

Analyze the following verbatim recording of this family therapy session. In making your analysis, refer to activity 50, "Guide to Interaction Process Analysis."

The James family was referred for counseling by an agency for retarded children with whom the family has contact. Mrs. James had expressed concern about the future of the marriage and the welfare of her children because of the conflict between her and her husband around matters of discipline. She believed the problem to be a result of his verbal abuse of her and his physical abuse of the children. Mr. James was an angry, rigid, and extremely suspicious man who believed that their problems arose from his wife's attitude toward his authority and her refusal to have a sexual relationship with him. Shortly after the second therapy session with the marital couple, Mr. James moved out of the house. Within a few more weeks, he had severed direct communication with all members of the family.

The family members are:

Dave James, the father, thirty-five years old. Three years ago he injured his back and was no longer able to continue his work as a landscape gardener. His behavior toward the children, especially the two boys, has become more violent since this time. He now works as a mail sorter.

Nancy James, thirty-four, the mother and housewife. She is a high school graduate who has not worked outside of the home since her marriage.

Jeff, the twelve-year-old son. He is a sixth-grade student who was held back in school one year for underachievement. Almost immediately after his father's departure from the home, Jeff's school work began to improve. He is not developmentally disabled.

Jimmy, the eight-year-old son. He is a second-grader, also held back one year for underachievement.

Karen, the seven-year-old daughter. She is in first grade and, like her brothers, was held back one year for underachievement.

Cora, the four-year-old daughter. She is severely developmentally disabled and requires total care. She lives at home.

This is the first session with the family and without the father. The nurse has arranged to come to the James house.

Interaction Process Analysis

INTERACTION (VERBAL AND NONVERBAL)	NURSE-CENTERED ANALYSIS	CLIENT-CENTERED ANALYSIS
(When the nurse arrived, Nancy looked quite tired and bedraggled but the house was neat and clean. Jeff was sitting at the dining room table doing homework. When the nurse invited him to join the group, he said he was much too busy. The nurse sat down on the living room couch, and the children milled about the room. Nancy also sat on the couch. The nurse showed them the tape recorder.)		
Nurse: Do you know what this is?		
Jimmy: See! I told you, Mom!		
Nancy: Tell the lady what you told me, Jimmy.		
Jimmy: I knew she'd have a tape recorder.		
Nancy: Well, go on!		
Jimmy (somewhat reluctantly): I told Mom you'd tape us and then let Dad hear it.		
(The nurse then explained the terms of confidentiality very clearly and told why she liked to use a tape recorder during a family meeting. She explained that after reviewing the tape she would erase it. The family		

INTERACTION (VERBAL AND NONVERBAL)	NURSE-CENTERED ANALYSIS	CLIENT-CENTERED ANALYSIS
seemed satisfied with this.)		
Nurse: I've already told you who I am and what I do. What I'd like to do now is hear from all of you about what you think is happening in your family?		
Karen: I think it's all wrong.		
Nurse: You think it's all wrong?		
Jimmy (very carefully enunciating): He's mixed up in the head. Right, Jeff?		
Karen: Yeah, he's blaming it all on Mommy, and it ain't true. He's doing . . .		
Jimmy (interrupts): Yeah, he's making up stuff.		
Nurse: Wait—wait. Let's try and set up a rule for our meetings. If someone is talking, let's wait until they're finished. Everyone will get a chance to talk.		
Jimmy: You mean raise our hand?		
Nurse: No. But if Karen is talking, wait until she is finished before you talk. Now, Karen, you were saying Dad is blaming everything on Mom, and it's all wrong.		
Karen: Yeah. And, he's hitting us too hard. He's hitting us in the head and it might		

INTERACTION (VERBAL AND NONVERBAL)	NURSE-CENTERED ANALYSIS	CLIENT-CENTERED ANALYSIS
damage our head. That ain't right to hit us in the face or the head.		
Jimmy: For one thing, he gave me a black eye already, and—this is kinda funny—my father pushed Jeff into the window (laughs).		
Nurse: What do you mean?		
Jimmy and Karen (talking at once): The big window in Jeff's room got broken.		
(Jimmy got up to demonstrate how his father pushed Jeff into the window, breaking it.)		
Nurse: You really think that's funny?		
Jimmy: No, not when it happened.		
Karen (speaking at the same time): No.		
Nurse: I don't see it as funny either.		
Jimmy: He says he believes in violence.		
Nurse: Is that the word he used?		
Jimmy: Yeah. He believes in violence. He says if you go out and play, and if anyone picks on you, break his jaw, and then go home, do your work, watch TV, and maybe play outside,		

INTERACTION (VERBAL AND NONVERBAL)	NURSE-CENTERED ANALYSIS	CLIENT-CENTERED ANALYSIS
and then go to bed. That's the way the day is supposed to go. . . . And working. . . . One little thing that Jeff and I do wrong, like take out the garbage, he smacks us. We go flying. Nurse: Gee, I wonder how you can take out the garbage wrong. Jimmy: He says there is only one way to do things—his way. Nurse: Do you believe there is only one way to do things? Jimmy and Karen: No. Karen: Plus, one night, um, um, you know, I didn't hear my mother cause I couldn't hear right and he kept smacking me until I did hear right. Like I was just sitting there eating my egg and my Mom was talking to me, but I didn't hear her. He screamed at me and kept hitting. Jimmy: Yeah. There's not one day that he doesn't smack me. I do something wrong, and he smacks me. Nurse: What kinds of things do you do wrong? Jimmy: He thinks when I come down the street, I stare at him and stuff. He thinks I'm a jerk. He's the jerk! I gotta tell you something: me and Karen were laying down watching TV like this (demonstrates how they		

INTERACTION (VERBAL AND NONVERBAL)	NURSE-CENTERED ANALYSIS	CLIENT-CENTERED ANALYSIS
were lying on the floor), just watching TV happily, and he comes along, kicks me and Karen in the back for no reason. "Get out of the way" (gruffly imitates father).		
Karen: Yeah, and we didn't even see him.		
Jimmy: Bam! "Get out of the way!"		
Karen: Then he kicked me in the spine and that really hurt.		
Nurse: Wow, how does that make you feel?		
Karen: I feel terrible.		
Jimmy: When I get bigger, oh, man! He's going to have a busted jaw. I'm going to get him back.		
Jeff (cries out): I'll smash him!		
Nurse: What was that, Jeff?		
Jeff: I didn't say anything. (He appeared to be quite busy with his work.)		
(Nancy took Cora upstairs and put her to bed, while the other children continued to talk. The nurse generally kept the talk on a superficial level, because she wanted Nancy present when the children were ventilating their feelings and experiences with their father. When Nancy returned, the nurse encouraged		

INTERACTION (VERBAL AND NONVERBAL)	NURSE-CENTERED ANALYSIS	CLIENT-CENTERED ANALYSIS
them to continue discussing their feelings about their father.)		
Karen: Well, the first time he left, I cried and cried. I couldn't stop. It just went on and on. But, you know, now it's better. It's so much better since he's gone.		
Jimmy: Yeah. Me and Jeff used to listen to him holler at Mom about her "games." He used to say that Mom was playing bedtime games.		
Nurse: Boy, sounds like you kids know a lot about what was going on between Mom and Dad.		
Jimmy: Sure we do.		
Karen (simultaneously): We're in the family.		
Nurse: Nancy, did you know that Karen and Jimmy were aware of the problems between you and Dave?		
Nancy (stammering): Well, I, I knew they knew something, but I guess not really so much.		
Jimmy: In the middle of the day, he screamed at Mom, and the screen door was open. And he used to smack Jeff right out in the open. He smacks me out in the open, and everybody stares.		
Karen: And you know what?		

INTERACTION (VERBAL AND NONVERBAL)	NURSE-CENTERED ANALYSIS	CLIENT-CENTERED ANALYSIS
Daddy pushed Mommy into the bushes one time. Nurse: Sounds like some pretty scary things have been happening here. Karen: Yeah. You should love your children. You should treat them right. When you have a life like this, you can't teach your children nothing. When you have problems, you can't do nothing. Jimmy: I know. Nurse: An example would help me get a clearer picture of what you mean. Karen: I mean when they're screaming at each other, I can't do nothing. I can't even play a game. It gets so scary. Jimmy: The other night we watched that movie about that man that beat his wife, and he threw the boy across the room. And then the lady lied about it. Boy, she shouldn't have lied about it. *I would not stick up for him!* (Said with emphasis.) (Jeff at this began to join the conversation, from the dining room, adding comments particularly of hate and vengeance toward the father.) Jeff: Dad is just like his own father, [the children's grandfather]. Mean and nasty.		

INTERACTION (VERBAL AND NONVERBAL)	NURSE-CENTERED ANALYSIS	CLIENT-CENTERED ANALYSIS
I know because my grandmother told me so. (The children began to talk among themselves, trying to think of possible explanations for their father's behavior. Jimmy felt that his father must have had high blood pressure to act the way he did. Jeff became very interested at this point.) Jeff (from dining room): It wouldn't make any difference what Dad did. He could go to the best psychiatrist in the world, but he will *never* change. Jimmy: He used to yell at her all the time because she wouldn't go dancing. Karen: Yeah. She ain't interested in that. That's crazy. Nurse: She isn't interested in what? Karen: Sex. Nurse: I wonder. Is that true, Mom? Karen (quite surprised): Are you? Nancy (laughs and then replies): Well, sure I am. Sex is an important part of a good relationship between a man and a woman. Jimmy: And Dad thinks me and Jeff are homosexuals. He said he caught me and Jeff fagging		

INTERACTION (VERBAL AND NONVERBAL)	NURSE-CENTERED ANALYSIS	CLIENT-CENTERED ANALYSIS
off. He's crazy—that ain't true. Nurse: You know what? I see you smiling, but I have a feeling you're not really smiling underneath. Jimmy: Not really, no! Man, he has no reason to say that. That's not true. He has no right to say that. (The discussion continued with more and more disclosures of beatings, hurts, and humiliations. Jeff joined in more and more. After about forty-five minutes, he left his work in the dining room to join the family in the living room.)		

TO THE OWNER OF THIS BOOK:

We hope that you have found *Psychosocial Nursing Concepts: An Activity Book, 3rd Edition*, a thought-provoking and enjoyable experience. We invite you to share your experiences in using this book with us so that your comments and suggestions will help to make it a better book for future editions. Fold as shown on back of this page. No postage is necessary.

School: _____

Location: _____

Instructor's Name: _____

1. What did you like most about *Psychosocial Nursing Concepts: An Activity Book*?

2. What did you like least?

3. If it was up to you, how would you like to see this book changed?

4. In what way has this book affected your attitudes and behaviors?

5. In the space below or in a separate letter please feel free to make any additional comments about this book that you'd like to.

Best wishes,

Holly Skodol Wilson and Carol Ren Kneisl

Optional:

Name: _____ Date: _____

Address: _____